Contents

PREFACE   xi

EXECUTIVE SUMMARY   1

1 INTRODUCTION   17
   The Context: Behavioral and Social Sciences at the
       National Institutes of Health, 18
   The Charge to the Committee, 19
   The Integrative Approach to Health, 21
   Key Influences on Pathways to Health, 22

2 PREDISEASE PATHWAYS   25
   Cumulative Physiological Risk, 26
   Characterizing Predisease Pathways, 28
   Connecting Predisease Pathways to Cumulative
       Physiological Risk, 39
   Recommendations, 40

3 POSITIVE HEALTH: RESILIENCE, RECOVERY, PRIMARY
   PREVENTION, AND HEALTH PROMOTION   45
   Resilience and Resistance to Disease: Who Stays Well and Why?, 47
   Recovery and Differential Survival Processes, 49
   Advancing the Science of Primary Prevention, 51
   New Directions in Positive Health Promotion, 54

Positive Health and the Council of Public Representatives, 56
Recommendations, 57

4   ENVIRONMENTALLY INDUCED GENE EXPRESSION   63
    Genes Expression and Prenatal Development, 64
    Personal Ties and Gene Expression in Midlife, 65
    Animal Models and the Consequences of Mother-Child
        Interactions, 66
    Intergenerational Transmission of Behavior, 67
    Plasticity of Genetic Trajectories, 68
    Whole-Genome Analyses, 69
    Recommendations, 70

5   PERSONAL TIES   73
    The Centrality of Personal Ties, 73
    Personal Ties and Gene Expression, 77
    Personal Ties and Brain Function and Structure, 78
    Personal Ties and Neuroimmunological Activity, 79
    Personal Ties and Infectious Disease, 81
        Social Relational Routes to Health, 82
    Recommendations, 84

6   COLLECTIVE PROPERTIES AND HEALTHY
    COMMUNITIES   91
    Community Contexts and Multilevel Research, 92
    Experimental Evidence, 93
    Mechanisms, 94
    Methodological Challenges and Research Priorities, 95
    Interactions of Individual and Collective Properties, 97
    Other Social Contexts, 97
    Recommendations, 98

7   THE INFLUENCE OF INEQUALITY ON HEALTH
    OUTCOMES   100
    Socioeconomic Status and Health, 100
    Racial and Ethnic Inequality and Discrimination, 106
    Recommendations, 111

8   POPULATION PERSPECTIVES: UNDERSTANDING
    HEALTH TRENDS AND EVALUATING THE HEALTH
    CARE SYSTEM   118
    Time Trends and Spatial Variation in Population Health, 118
    Accounting for Macro-Level Health Patterns, 130

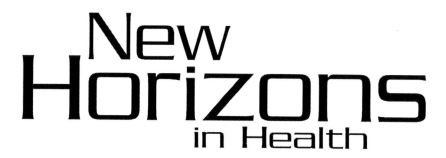

New Horizons in Health

in Health

An Integrative Approach

Committee on Future Directions for Behavioral and Social
Sciences Research at the National Institutes of Health

Burton H. Singer and Carol D. Ryff, *editors*

Board on Behavioral, Cognitive, and Sensory Sciences

Commission on Behavioral and Social Sciences and Education
National Research Council

NATIONAL ACADEMY PRESS
Washington, D.C.

NATIONAL ACADEMY PRESS   2101 Constitution Avenue, N.W.   Washington, D.C.   20418

NOTICE: The project that is the subject of this report was approved by the Governing Board of the National Research Council, whose members are drawn from the councils of the National Academy of Sciences, the National Academy of Engineering, and the Institute of Medicine. The members of the committee responsible for the report were chosen for their special competences and with regard for appropriate balance.

The study was supported by Grant No. N01-OD-4-2139, #56, between the National Academy of Sciences and the U.S. Department of Health and Human Services. Any opinions, findings, conclusions, or recommendations expressed in this publication are those of the author(s) and do not necessarily reflect the views of the organizations or agencies that provided support for this project.

Library of Congress Cataloging-in-Publication Data

National Research Council (U.S.). Committee on Future Directions for Behavioral and Social Sciences Research at the National Institutes of Health.
   New horizons in health : an integrative approach / Committee on Future Directions for Behavioral and Social Sciences Research at the National Institutes of Health, Board on Behavioral, Cognitive, and Sensory Sciences, Commission on Behavioral and Social Sciences and Education, National Research Council ; Burton H. Singer and Carol D. Ryff, editors.
      p. cm.
Includes bibliographical references and index.
   ISBN 0-309-07296-4 (pbk.)
   1. Health promotion—United States. 2. Medicine, Preventive—United States. 3. Health planning—United States. 4. Integrated delivery of health care—United States. I. Singer, Burton H. II. Ryff, Carol D. III. Title.
   RA394 .N365 2001
   613'.0973—dc21
                                        00-012474

Additional copies of this report are available from National Academy Press, 2101 Constitution Avenue, N.W., Lockbox 285, Washington, D.C. 20418.

Call (800) 624-6242 or (202) 334-3313 (in the Washington metropolitan area).

This report is also available online at http://www.nap.edu.

Suggested citation: National Research Council. 2001. *New Horizons in Health: An Integrative Approach*. Committee on Future Directions for Behavioral and Social Sciences Research at the National Institutes of Health, Singer BH, Ryff CD, eds. (Washington, DC: National Academy Press).

Printed in the United States of America

THE NATIONAL ACADEMIES

National Academy of Sciences
National Academy of Engineering
Institute of Medicine
National Research Council

The **National Academy of Sciences** is a private, nonprofit, self-perpetuating society of distinguished scholars engaged in scientific and engineering research, dedicated to the furtherance of science and technology and to their use for the general welfare. Upon the authority of the charter granted to it by the Congress in 1863, the Academy has a mandate that requires it to advise the federal government on scientific and technical matters. Dr. Bruce M. Alberts is president of the National Academy of Sciences.

The **National Academy of Engineering** was established in 1964, under the charter of the National Academy of Sciences, as a parallel organization of outstanding engineers. It is autonomous in its administration and in the selection of its members, sharing with the National Academy of Sciences the responsibility for advising the federal government. The National Academy of Engineering also sponsors engineering programs aimed at meeting national needs, encourages education and research, and recognizes the superior achievements of engineers. Dr. William A. Wulf is president of the National Academy of Engineering.

The **Institute of Medicine** was established in 1970 by the National Academy of Sciences to secure the services of eminent members of appropriate professions in the examination of policy matters pertaining to the health of the public. The Institute acts under the responsibility given to the National Academy of Sciences by its congressional charter to be an adviser to the federal government and, upon its own initiative, to identify issues of medical care, research, and education. Dr. Kenneth I. Shine is president of the Institute of Medicine.

The **National Research Council** was organized by the National Academy of Sciences in 1916 to associate the broad community of science and technology with the Academy's purposes of furthering knowledge and advising the federal government. Functioning in accordance with general policies determined by the Academy, the Council has become the principal operating agency of both the National Academy of Sciences and the National Academy of Engineering in providing services to the government, the public, and the scientific and engineering communities. The Council is administered jointly by both Academies and the Institute of Medicine. Dr. Bruce M. Alberts and Dr. William A. Wulf are chairman and vice chairman, respectively, of the National Research Council.

Health and the Macroeconomy, 135
The Health Care System, 137
Future Directions in Population Surveys, 142
Recommendations, 143

9   INTERVENTIONS   148
Experience with Interventions, 150
Key Trends, 155
Future Research Needs and Directions, 157
Recommendations, 159

10 METHODOLOGY PRIORITIES   164
Characterizing Pathways, 165
Advancing the Understanding of Biological Mechanisms, 170
Methods of Data Analysis, 175
Design and Evaluation of Intervention Programs, 178
Recommendations, 179

11 RESEARCH INFRASTRUCTURE   184
High Priority Human and Animal Populations, 184
Clinical Research Centers, 186
Communities and Interventions, 187
Training, 188
Recommendations, 188

BIOGRAPHICAL SKETCHES   190

INDEX   197

Preface

In 1999, Norman Anderson, director of the Office of Behavioral and Social Sciences Research (OBSSR) of the National Institutes of Health (NIH), asked the National Research Council (NRC) to form a committee that could develop a research plan to guide NIH in supporting areas of high priority in the behavioral and social sciences.

Suggestions for committee membership came from numerous sources, including the NRC Board on Behavioral, Cognitive, and Sensory Sciences, OBSSR and the NIH institutes, and members of the Commission on Behavioral and Social Sciences and Education (CBASSE). This process, representing input from multiple sources, culminated in a committee whose membership consisted of 15 scientists (named at the beginning of this volume) with diverse backgrounds and perspectives in the biomedical and social behavioral fields as well as extensive experience reaching across the scientific disciplines. It is a notable strength of the committee that selection of its members was weighted on the side of those who have established track records in multidisciplinary research and are at the forefront of the biobehavioral interface in current science. It is therefore not surprising that a majority had previous exposure to multidisciplinary efforts such as the research networks of the John D. and Catherine T. MacArthur Foundation. These networks have played pivotal roles in nurturing integrative science over the last 15 years by bringing together teams of investigators from diverse fields to work together on targeted agendas. This background to the committee membership is relevant because bringing the behavioral and social sciences more strongly and visibly into the full panorama of health research at the NIH is dependent on building bridges across the scientific disciplines.

The committee met four times between May 1999 and February 2000. After reviewing the charge from OBSSR and NRC procedures for preparing such a report, the committee planned a workshop to solicit information and advice from representatives of each of the NIH institutes and the NIH director's Council of Public Representatives (COPR) regarding topics the committee needed to consider in its deliberations. Second, the workshop was to be a forum for an exchange of views between members of the committee and representatives of the institutes concerning useful ways to respond to the committee's charge.

At the workshop, the committee listened to presentations by representatives of nearly all institutes of NIH. They spoke about ongoing programs in the behavioral and social sciences and provided their views of promising future directions. These presentations were lucid, informative, and especially helpful to the committee regarding the scope of extant social behavioral work as well as for identifying future venues for biobehavioral integration. After the workshop, the committee worked for several months to shape and develop its report.

In addition to the workshop presentations, valuable input to the committee was also provided by Melanie Dreher, dean of the School of Nursing at the University of Iowa, who was the liaison with the COPR. Authorized by Congress, the COPR is charged with consulting, advising, and making recommendations to the NIH on issues of development of programmatic priorities. The COPR also has the task of enhancing public participation in NIH activities, increasing public understanding of NIH and its programs, and bringing important matters of public interest forward for discussion in public settings. COPR input to the committee played an important role in shaping the research priorities put forward in this report. Benefiting the health of the public is central to the proposed integrative approach, and an entire chapter of this report is focused on positive health promotion, a key theme from the COPR.

This report was reviewed in draft form by individuals chosen for their diverse perspectives and technical expertise, in accordance with procedures approved by the NRC's Report Review Committee. The purpose of this independent review is to provide candid and critical comments that will assist the institution in making its published report as sound as possible and to ensure that the report meets institutional standards for objectivity, evidence, and responsiveness to the study charge. The review comments and draft manuscript remain confidential to protect the integrity of the deliberative process. We wish to thank the following individuals for their review of this report: Nancy E. Adler, Department of Psychiatry and Pediatrics, Center for Health and Community, University of California, San Francisco;

Bernard J. Carroll, Pacific Behavioral Research Foundation, Carmel, California; David S. Cordray, Institute for Public Policy Studies, Vanderbilt University; Karen Emmons, Dana Farber Cancer Institute, Boston, Massachusetts; Victor R. Fuchs, Department of Economics, Stanford University (emeritus); Beatrix Hamburg, Department of Psychiatry, Cornell University Medical College; E.A. Hammel, Department of Demography, University of California, Berkeley; James House, Institute of Social Research, University of Michigan; Stephen Manuck, Department of Psychology, University of Pittsburgh; Elissa L. Newport, Department of Brain and Cognitive Sciences, University of Rochester; and Robert Sapolsky, Department of Biological Sciences, Stanford University.

Although the reviewers listed above provided many constructive comments and suggestions, they were not asked to endorse the conclusions or recommendations nor did they see the final draft of the report before its release. The review of this report was overseen by Neil Smelser, Center for Advanced Study in the Behavioral Sciences, Stanford, California, and David R. Challoner, Institute for Science and Health Policy, University of Florida. Appointed by the Commission on Behavioral and Social Sciences and Education and the NRC's Report Review Committee, respectively, they were responsible for making certain that an independent examination of this report was carried out in accordance with institutional procedures and that all review comments were carefully considered. Responsibility for the final content of this report rests entirely with the authoring committee and the institution.

We would especially like to thank Barbara Boyle Torrey, executive director of the Commission on Behavioral and Social Sciences and Education, for sustained support, encouragement, and guidance throughout the preparation of this report. Help from NRC staff has also been valuable. We would like to thank representatives of the NIH institutes, who made presentations to the committee about their programs in social and behavioral science research. Finally, we would like to again thank Melanie Dreher of COPR for identifying health issues and concerns from the general public that need to be factored into future priorities about research and practice.

Burton H. Singer, *Chair and Coeditor*
Carol D. Ryff, *Coeditor*
Committee on Future Directions for
Behavioral and Social Sciences Research at the
National Institutes of Health

Executive Summary

T his report identifies a broad domain of questions at the interface of social, behavioral, and biomedical sciences, whose resolution could lead to major improvements in the health of the U.S. population. In creating a vision of future directions, the committee emphasized research priorities that cut across institute boundaries at the National Institutes of Health (NIH), thereby underscoring the broad significance of behavioral and social science research for multiple disease outcomes as well as health promotion. The background criteria guiding the development of priorities were that they should represent areas of great scientific opportunity and address pressing health problems, including health concerns of the general public. A leitmotiv of the corpus of opportunities identified in this report is that they cannot be addressed successfully by either the biomedical sciences or the behavioral and social sciences acting alone. Greater integration of health research and practice across these broad domains is essential to implement the committee's recommendations.

Behavioral and social science research has a long history at NIH. For example, the National Heart Institute, predecessor of the National Heart, Lung, and Blood Institute, was founded in 1948 and funded its first behavioral science research grant in 1955, focused on psychological factors related to high blood pressure and coronary heart disease. The National Cancer Institute, established by Congress in 1937, has an extensive behavioral research program emphasizing cancer prevention and control. The historical roots of this broad agenda reside in the mandates of the National Cancer Act passed by Congress in 1971. More generally, many of the institutes have longstanding and well-developed behavioral and social science programs. Trans-institute initiatives with linkages to basic biology are also appearing with increasing frequency, such as recent requests for proposals on socioeconomic status and health and the establishment of mind/body centers.

At the same time, the behavioral and social sciences have limited presence at some institutes or are seen as peripheral to primary agendas. Also when considered, behavioral, psychological, and social priorities are sometimes restricted to a narrow focus on their role as risk factors for particular disease outcomes. A central message of this report is that behavioral and psychosocial processes have broader significance and are fundamental to a comprehensive understanding of disease etiology as well as to promotion of health and well-being.

Building on recognition of these prior strengths and weaknesses, the Committee on Future Directions for Behavioral and Social Sciences Research at NIH embarked on its task. The committee was created under the Board on Behavioral, Cognitive, and Sensory Sciences of the National Research Council. It was established via a request by the Office of Behavioral and Social Sciences Research (OBSSR) to the NRC to evaluate the potential contributions of behavioral and social science research to the mission of NIH and to develop research priorities that support and complement the work of the institutes.

The committee's deliberations regarding investigations that would satisfy the complementary demands of high scientific payoff and response to pressing health concerns led to the identification of 10 thematic priorities. An overarching theme is a focus on multiple pathways to diverse health outcomes. Pathway characterizations integrate information from the molecular and cellular level with psychosocial and community levels and thereby represent routes to deeper understanding of disease etiology as well as resilience in the face of adversity. The mechanisms underlying racial, ethnic, and social inequalities in health also cannot be fully understood without integrated pathway characterizations. Pathway approaches also provide a comprehensive approach to health-promoting interventions. Early intervention and prevention have societal-level payoff in increasing active life expectancy and delaying the age of onset of disabilities. At the same time, the integrated pathway approach affords the knowledge base for more individualized forms of health care.

This report describes in detail the 10 thematic priorities highlighted below. Specific recommendations for research opportunities following from each of them are briefly outlined in this Executive Summary. These recommendations are elaborated at the conclusion of the individual chapters that follow. In addition to the thematic priorities, one overarching recommendation is put forth: the need to institutionalize the integrative approach at NIH.

THEMATIC PRIORITIES

The committee recommends 10 priority areas for research investment to integrate the behavioral, social, and biomedical sciences at the National Institutes of Health:

1. Predisease pathways—identify early and long-term biological, behavioral, psychological, and social precursors to disease;
2. Positive health—identify biological, behavioral, and psychosocial factors that contribute to resilience, disease resistance, and wellness;
3. Gene expression—understand environmentally induced gene expression and its connection to positive and negative health outcomes;
4. Personal ties—explicate the mechanisms by which proximal social interactions influence health and disease outcomes;
5. Healthy communities—identify the collective properties of social and physical environments that influence health and disease outcomes;
6. Inequality—clarify the mechanisms through which socioeconomic hierarchies, racism, discrimination, and stigmatization influence health and disease outcomes;
7. Population health—understand macro-level trends in health status and evaluate the performance of the health care system;
8. Interventions—expand the scope and effectiveness of strategies for social and behavioral interventions to improve health;
9. Methodology—develop new measurement techniques and study designs to link information across levels of analysis (molecular, cellular, behavioral, psychosocial, community) and across time;
10. Infrastructure—establish ways to maintain long-term study populations and to train scientists to integrate health-related knowledge across multiple disciplines.

The scope of the priorities is expansive, with each encompassing wide areas of research. Some represent more individual-level phenomena, while others deal with macro-level (e.g., population) issues. The sections that follow describe the thematic priorities and identify the principal recommendations associated with them.

1. Predisease Pathways

We use the term "predisease pathway" to describe the biological influences (e.g., genetic factors, endocrine and immune factors) and related links to behavioral, psychological, and social influences that precede morbidity and mortality. A primary message is the need to assess precursors to disease at points more distant temporally than has been examined in most previous research. Equally important is the need to study the biological, behavioral, psychological, and social precursors to disease *simultaneously*. Wider time horizons are required to understand early antecedents to later risk factors as well as the long-term etiological processes involved in multiple disease outcomes. Predisease pathways thus include a broad array of factors that affect the individual from conception (or before) through development and adulthood into later life. Illustrative influences include prenatal and early risk factors, along with a diverse array of psychological factors (e.g., control and efficacy, temperament, optimism, cognitive states, emotion regulation), behavioral factors (e.g., diet, exercise, smoking, alcohol consumption, drug abuse, sexual activity), and familial and environmental influences (e.g., social ties and support, family stress, work conditions, community supports).

Building on the guiding theme of integrative research, there is need to assess physiological risk across multiple systems simultaneously. Repeated or continuous exposure to challenge or chronic underexposure and social isolation disrupts basic biological regulatory processes central to the maintenance of homeostasis and health. When exposed to challenge at vulnerable times (e.g., during early stages of pre- and postnatal development) or repeatedly during later periods of life, multiple physiological responses may operate outside of normal ranges. Over time, this exacts wear and tear—i.e., cumulative physiological risk—on humans and animals. Operationalization of culmulative risk across systems and across time is an important aspect of characterizing predisease pathways. Illustrating needed research in this direction are emerging studies of allostatic load, a preliminary formulation of cumulative physiological risk. Also critical is the need to track the unfolding interactions between genetic factors and environmental influences over time.

A basic research initiative throughout the NIH institutes should be focused on predisease pathways, including the following topics:

• identification of early markers of predisease states;
• examination of their genetic and environmental origins through animal and human studies;
• identification of behavioral risk factors in the exacerbation or amelioration of predisease pathways;
• prioritization of experimental and longitudinal research to chart these trajectories across the life span; studies should consider biological, behavioral, psychological, and social precursors to disease simultaneously;
• focus on the mechanisms by which genetic influences, early life experiences, and behavioral and psychosocial risk factors across the life span

interact, leading to accumulating physiological risk and a broad range of disease outcomes.

2. Positive Health

A critical counterpoint to understanding pathways to disease is the need to advance knowledge of positive health, which includes not only the absence of illness but also the presence of wellness. Understanding the etiology and promotion of positive health outcomes requires expanded scientific agendas on resilience and resistance to disease processes as well as recovery and differential survival from illness. Greater emphasis must be given to primary prevention and positive health promotion as routes to extending disability-free years for larger segments of the population. Sustaining or regaining optimal health requires a focus on behavioral (e.g., positive health practices), psychological (e.g., optimism, purpose, mastery, positive affect, religion/spirituality), social (e.g., relational affect and intimacy, emotional support), and environmental (e.g., positive work settings, supportive community programs) factors. Explicating the biological substrates of these components and their role in delaying the onset of morbidity and mortality represent major research opportunities of the future.

To advance the positive health agenda, NIH should:

• target new research on the neurobiological mechanisms (e.g., allostasis—variation in the internal milieu to meet external demands, balance of anabolic and catabolic systems, neurogenesis and expression of neurotrophins) through which positive behavioral and psychosocial factors (e.g., exercise, enriched environments, quality social relationships, psychological well-being) influence health;

• establish new priorities focused on the etiology (at genetic, behavioral, environmental levels) of disease resistance, particularly in contexts of known risk;

• increase support for the study of the protective resources (optimism, meaning and purpose, social and emotional support, and related neurobiological mechanisms) that promote recovery and increased survival rates;

• initiate new investigations that will advance knowledge of resilience in the face of life adversity, giving particular emphasis to longitudinal studies;

• advance the science of primary prevention, giving particular attention to overcoming persistent maladaptive behaviors (e.g., drinking, smoking, sedentary lifestyles, poor stress management);

• develop new population-based initiatives, implemented at local community levels, that promote health via the teaching of positive life practices and the provision of environmental supports to sustain them.

3. Environmentally Induced Gene Expression

In-depth understanding of pathways to disease and preservation of good health necessitates the study of environmentally induced gene expression. Recent research has revealed that specific genes can be expressed at different points in an organism's life. Whether a particular gene is expressed and the degree to which it is expressed depend strongly on the environmental conditions experienced by the organism. Such gene expression is implicated in both positive and negative health effects.

Animal studies have been and will continue to be the main route to achieving deeper understanding of the mechanisms of gene expression. Environmental influences on gene expression in animal models include short-term early life influences (e.g., release of placental growth hormone, response to maternal stress hormones) and long-term responses to environmental conditions (e.g., physiological consequences of nurturing). The recent availability of gene chip technology provides the capability to identify changes in gene expression in response to environmental manipulations.

NIH should support integrative research aimed at understanding the role of environmentally induced gene expression in disease etiology and promotion of health. This should include:

- studies that combine environmental manipulations with physiological and molecular assessments to provide refined understanding of conditions leading to dysfunction and, concomitantly, the mechanisms that preserve allostasis; investigation of connections between personal ties, the physical environment, and gene expression are particularly important;
- studies that explore in animal models the relationships between chronic stress, interactions among intervening systems (e.g., hypothalamic-pituitary-adrenal axis, autonomic nervous system, immune system and overall central nervous system control of these systems), gene expression, and health outcomes;
- initiation of studies using microarray chip technologies to monitor gene expression, associated with a broad range of environmental manipulations;
- development of animal housing facilities, particularly for rodents, that more closely approximate species-specific habitats.

4. Personal Ties

The preceding priorities (predisease pathways, positive health, and environmentally induced gene expression) all emphasize the importance of proximal social interactions. Survival of newborns depends on nurturance by others, and extensive lines of inquiry illustrate the centrality of social ties across the life course. A large body of epidemiological findings document the links between social relationships and mental and physical health outcomes, including mortality. Disruption of personal ties, loneliness, and conflictual interactions are key sources of stress, while supportive social connections and intimate relations are vital sources of emotional strength.

What is not well understood, however, are the connections between these realms of personal connection and gene expression, brain structure and function, neuroimmunological activity, and ultimate disease and health outcomes. Reflecting the focus on pathways, there is a pressing need to assess cumulative long-term relational profiles, particularly their emotional features, and link them to cumulative physiological profiles, such as allostatic load. In the extant literature, analyses also tend to focus on average responses and frequently relegate individual differences to error variance. Given the need to understand multiple pathways to diverse health outcomes, such individual differences should be treated as a crucible for theory construction and empirical testing.

NIH studies of the links between the social world and health should focus on the underlying and causal (including reciprocal) mechanisms in both animals and humans. The objective is to understand interrelationships between social interaction and correlative biological phenomena. This work should include:

- studies that explicate the links between social relationships and gene expression, brain structure and function, and neuroimmunological activity;
- investigations that assess how social ties influence health practices and behaviors;
- longitudinal studies that link cumulative social relational profiles with cumulative biological profiles;
- increased emphasis on the collection of biomarkers in epidemiological studies of social relationships and health;
- extensions of traditional laboratory studies to include experience sampling methodologies and corresponding ambulatory neurobiological assessments;
- multilevel integrative studies working at the interface of social interaction, emotion, and brain activity and downstream endocrinological and immunological processes.

5. Healthy Communities

The preceding emphasis on social environments reflects primarily individual-level influences and processes. This report underscores the importance of conducting more extensive research on the collective properties of social environments. This requires treating the community as a unit of analysis in its own right. Neighborhoods can be characterized by levels of poverty, unemployment, residential instability, housing characteristics, and racial/ethnic mix as well as by rates of crime, mental illness, morbidity, and mortality. Research shows that even when individual attributes and behaviors are taken into account, there are further influences on health outcomes following from collective community properties. Social processes in these collective sources of influence that require investigation include such phenomena as social cohesion, subcultures of violence, and informal social controls. Integrating collective properties into ongoing health research will also require attending to interactions between individual- and community-level variables. Future work in this area also depends on the resolution of multiple methodological challenges (e.g., dealing with nested levels of aggregation, simultaneity bias, and differential selection).

A possible model for developing standardized indicators of the health of communities is the Sustainable Seattle project. A standardized approach to assessment of community health would eventually allow cities and neighborhoods to evaluate how well they are doing in responding to their own health-related goals and in comparison with other cities and neighborhoods.

Adding contextual information to ongoing studies (e.g., Current Population Survey, Panel Study of Income Dynamics) is a relatively economical way to begin making connections between individual- and community-level variables. A particularly important opportunity associated with such data augmentation is the unprecedented change in social environments occurring across many urban communities in the United States as a result of devolving public housing. Especially in large cities, families are being relocated and entire housing projects are being dispersed. The quasi-experimental nature of these changes provides opportunities to learn about the connection between health outcomes and environmental change.

NIH-supported research on healthy communities should include the following kinds of work:

- development of a benchmark assessment (standardized approach) of the collective health of communities;
- selection of and support for longitudinal studies that target data augmentation and multilevel analysis, with a particular focus on person-environment interactions;
- investigation of contextual factors (e.g., cohesion, informal social control, physical disorder, local support networks) as mediators of health or disease outcomes;

• design of prevention strategies to promote aggregate-level health by changing social and community environments (e.g., regulation of smoking in public places, taxation policies).

6. Inequality and Health Outcomes

Human and animal studies show that position in social hierarchies influences morbidity and mortality. A recent trans-institute initiative on socioeconomic status and health seeks to understand how the inverse associations between indicators of socioeconomic position and a wide array of health outcomes come about. Further advances in this area must incorporate both individual-level variables and collective properties of community environments. In addition, programs of study are needed on the role of socioeconomic hierarchies in predisease pathways, which encompass behavioral, psychosocial, and environmental factors as well as underlying biological mechanisms.

Disparities in health following from ethnic/racial status and related experiences of discrimination, racism, and stigmatization must be key priorities under the broader rubric of social inequalities. There is also a pressing need to study cumulative experience along pathways to adverse health outcomes via long-term tracking of chronic features of economic, educational, and racial/ethnic disadvantage. It is clear that observed variations in health are not driven simply by expenditures on medical care or by absolute levels of affluence. What is needed are systematic efforts to characterize health-relevant aspects of social environments. For example, mortality rates of blacks and whites are elevated in cities high on indices of racial residential segregation, but the possible intervening mechanisms between place of residence and health status are unknown. The concept of cumulative physiological risk provides a useful framework for tracing pathways from environmental exposures to changes in health status.

Moving beyond the current NIH initiatives on socioeconomic status and health, the committee recommends the following foci of attention:

• characterization of behavioral and environmental risks associated with educational, economic, and occupational disparities;
• elaboration of the subjective experience of racism, discrimination, and stigmatization and their effects on behavior as well as their neurobiological substrates;
• assessment of health-related impacts of large-scale societal structures (e.g., racial segregation, economic discrimination, differential access to services and medical care);
• development of integrative longitudinal studies that connect socio-

economic-related risk factors to intervening biological systems and subsequent health outcomes;

   • identification of cultural strengths and health-enhancing resources resident in racial/ethnic groups and their role in accounting for resilience vis-à-vis socioeconomic inequality.

7. Population Health

Previously listed priorities on predisease pathways, positive health, and environmentally induced gene expression place strong emphasis on preventing disease and promoting well-being at levels proximal to the individual. Collective properties of communities and social inequalities in turn address health at intermediate levels of aggregation. At the highest macro-level is population health. This report emphasizes four population issues: (1) time trends and spatial variation in population health; (2) accounting for such trends, with particular emphasis given to social and behavioral factors; (3) understanding linkages between the macroeconomy and population health; and (4) evaluating the health care system. An important crosscutting issue between these topics and the preceding priorities is the need for multilevel analyses that link population health dynamics to behavioral, psychosocial, and environmental factors (at both individual and intermediate levels of aggregation).

Recently documented population changes include declining rates of disability among the elderly and the growing utilization of alternative medicine. These require a broad range of in-depth studies to understand their origins, such as the role of behavioral and psychosocial factors in accounting for declining later-life disabilities. In the case of alternative therapies, what is needed is an integrated biopsychosocial characterization of their mechanisms of action and clear indications of what works, for whom, and why. With regard to children, deeper understanding of the causes of asthma, the most common chronic disease of childhood, lies in the future. Although several NIH initiatives are currently in progress to address gaps in current knowledge, investigations are needed to integrate data and findings from these studies into a unified multilevel explanation of how asthma comes about. These examples illustrate the central challenge for population-level research, namely, to identify the most important factors that drive changes in population health and to clarify their impact on society at large.

Evaluating the health care system is also a key priority. Of central importance are studies that will clarify how health outcomes are affected by managed care and explain the many conflicting findings regarding the effectiveness of medical care. Increased support for research on reciprocal relationships between population health and the macroeconomy is also a priority.

The committee recommends that NIH support a broad-gauged set of initiatives that include the following specific topics:

• multilevel analyses necessary to advance rigorous explanations for the observed dynamics of the health of populations, giving particular emphasis to behavioral, psychosocial, and environmental influences on aggregate-level health changes;

• development of projection methodologies to provide defensible scenarios of how health changes will affect society in the future;

• conceptual and empirical research on the value of biomedical innovations and the way they affect the health care system.

8. Interventions

Numerous preventive and therapeutic interventions have been introduced over past decades to help people to live longer and improve their quality of life. Interventions that have been widely implemented and emphasize behavioral and social factors include those designed to decrease behaviors associated with health risk (e.g., alcohol or substance abuse, smoking) or increase behaviors associated with health promotion (e.g., exercise, dietary practices). A further category receiving increased attention are interventions aimed at facilitating effective coping with chronic conditions and life-threatening diseases. Less extensive as yet are programs focused on family and social network interventions.

Historically, most studies have focused on the assessment of single interventions. However, the success of multiple-intervention programs, targeted simultaneously at different life domains and physiological systems, calls for more broad-gauged approaches to program development. In particular, we emphasize the need for interventions targeted at multiple levels (e.g., individual, family, organizational, population) as well as being pertinent to large segments of the population, not just high-risk groups. At the organizational level, we underscore prior success with work site and school-based programs and emphasize their inclusion in community-level intervention packages. We also emphasize the need for dynamic interventions that are adaptive over time and thereby address changing personal, social, and environmental circumstances.

We recommend that NIH support a new generation of intervention studies with the following emphases:

• development of strategies for extending successful social and behavioral interventions to more heterogeneous populations, including those focused on prevention via early identification of persons at risk;

- promote research and interventions in health-related decision making, such as how individuals understand the content of health communications as well as manage their own health needs and risks;
- expansion of implementation and dissemination activities so as to reduce the gap between research progress and practice;
- development of an overall strategy for intervention research that integrates behavioral, psychosocial, and biomedical approaches and that spans multiple levels, from the individual to the societal;
- intervention research that capitalizes on new opportunities created by technological innovation.

9. Methodological Priorities

New measurement techniques and designs for both animal and human studies are necessary to build bridges that will link behavioral, psychological, and social levels of analysis to multiple levels of biology (organ systems, cellular, molecular). This broad purview underscores the need for methodologies that are responsive to the functioning of complex dynamical systems through time. To advance priorities on predisease pathways and positive health it is critically important to conduct longitudinal studies that measure multiple domains (e.g., behavioral, psychological, social, environmental) across time (e.g., early life influences, childhood and adolescence, adulthood, and old age). Parallel longitudinal requirements pertain to the biological mechanisms through which the above factors affect health outcomes. As such, longitudinal studies will increasingly require broad-based forms of data collection—social, behavioral, and biomedical.

Related to this general issue, the concept of cumulative physiological risk, illustrated with allostatic load, requires further refinement to better understand the cascade of internal events from optimal functioning of multiple systems to accumulating risk. Full understanding of predisease pathways will require operationalizations of cumulative multisystem risk that are suitable for infants, young children, and adolescents. The emphasis on pathways in this report also implies a need for statistical methodologies that can specify pathway trajectories, address nonlinearities in diverse indicators, and incorporate narratives as sources of data. Pertinent to the enlarged scope of intervention studies, greater understanding will be required of processes of voluntary self-selection in design and evaluation of complex multiple-component programs.

Specifically, we recommend that NIH support methodological initiatives in four broad areas:

1. refine the operationalization of cumulative physiological risk that takes explicit account of the internal cascade of events leading to risk across

multiple systems; ambulatory assessments and responses to transient challenges should be given consideration as potential components of improved measures of cumulative physiological risk;

2. develop and refine instruments for measuring positive psychosocial factors; this initiative is fundamental for characterizing pathways to positive health outcomes;

3. develop person-centered statistical methodologies to facilitate characterizations of predisease and positive health pathways that link behavioral, psychosocial, environmental, and biological levels of analysis;

4. develop design, implementation, and analysis strategies for multiple-component interventions where allowance is made for adaptive, dynamic tuning of the interventions to obtain optimal outcomes.

10. Research Infrastructure and Training

This report makes clear the need for sustained core support of human and animal populations that can be used to investigate integrated biopsychosocial pathways to diverse health outcomes (positive and negative). Relevant human populations include longitudinal survey and community samples. Relevant animal populations include free-ranging and laboratory colonies of numerous species. The much-needed integration of behavioral, psychological, social, and environmental conditions, along with biomedical factors, can be facilitated via additions to ongoing longitudinal studies as well as through development of new birth cohort samples. The domain of health promotion and primary disease prevention requires a selected set of communities and core populations within them to provide comprehensive multiple-level health information and to engage in complex community-wide intervention studies.

The multidisciplinary nature of all thematic priorities in this report underscores a critical and pervasive need for training initiatives to nurture, support, and sustain hybrid careers that transcend current disciplinary boundaries. NIH has had some success in fostering such careers. However, success in the integrative studies central to this report will require a new cadre of scientists facile in working across social, behavioral, and biomedical levels of analysis.

In light of these needs, NIH should provide core support for sustained infrastructure in two areas:

1. longitudinal survey populations, human communities, laboratory animal colonies, and free-ranging animal communities;

2. training initiatives to nurture and regularize the hybrid (multidisciplinary) careers of a new generation of scientists.

Any long-term plan for research should be adaptive and subject to regular reassessment. This would be most effectively accomplished with cross-institute strategic planning and trans-institute initiatives. It is our hope that this report provides NIH with the rationale to implement a wide-ranging and long-term commitment to integration of the behavioral, social, and biomedical sciences in pursuit of improving the health of the U.S. population. Our final recommendation pertains to this larger integrative task.

The Need to Institutionalize the Integrative Approach at NIH

The vision of research proposed in this report, with its focus on the unfolding interactions between genetic, behavioral, psychosocial, and environmental factors over time and its recurrent emphasis on multilevel analysis, highlights the need for greater cross-institute strategic planning and trans-institute research initiatives. The committee has not been asked and is in no position to make detailed recommendations regarding the structure of NIH. However, in our judgment, the success of an integrative research approach will require collaborative efforts of the entire NIH community of scientists—medical, biological, behavioral, and social. Both incentive structures and an institutional presence will greatly facilitate such collaborative strides. As a first step **the committee recommends that NIH create internal mechanisms for developing consensus on the most promising research opportunities within and across the thematic priorities as well as a locus for strategic planning for future trans-institute initiatives.**

Pathways to Health: A Vision for the Future

The committee received very useful input from the Council of Public Representatives (COPR). The COPR offers a public forum for discussing key NIH issues (e.g., priority setting, clinical trials, managed care, privacy and genetics, health disparities). COPR members review and advise on NIH priorities and thereby provide public input to NIH decisions. Its strong message to the committee was that NIH should do more to help people create and lead healthy lives. Many people perceive NIH as focused on curing disease rather than on promoting quality living, optimal families, supportive work environments, and healthy communities. The COPR also called for more information about how the general public can take more effective responsibility for its own health care. The thematic priorities in this report are very much a response to these messages from COPR. The priorities point toward multiple new directions at NIH that are intended to promote better health for ever larger segments of the U.S. population via deeper understanding of the interacting processes (biological, psychological, social, environmental) through which illness occurs or wellness is maintained. The ultimate payoff for the health of the public of the pathway focus emphasized throughout this report is prevention and health care strategies that are more effectively tailored and targeted to the set of circumstances confronting individuals, communities, and populations.

1

Introduction

Historically speaking, human health has been a tale of ever-shifting horizons. For much of the distant past, health was equivalent to short-term survival in the face of food scarcity, predators, and pestilence. With gains in agriculture, sanitation, and the growth of community, length of life was extended somewhat. Later, the scientific revolution transformed health into a biological realm that was primarily the purview of medical fields, at least in Western and economically developed cultures. The past century has witnessed dramatic gains in longevity, thanks to unprecedented advances in diagnosing, treating, and preventing disease, along with unimaginable gains in technology that facilitate understanding health at molecular, cellular, and genetic levels. Still, there remains significant distance to travel in the journey toward optimal human health. The horizon before us is one in which health encompasses not only the workings of biology, the brain, and the body but also the human mind, its thoughts and feelings, human actions and behavior, as well as the nature of social ties, friendships, family, and community life.

With this vision before us, we call for a new era of research and practice at the National Institutes of Health (NIH) that integrates biomedical and social behavioral fields of inquiry to promote the nation's health. Increasing evidence documents the role of behavioral, psychological, social, and environmental factors as causes of death. In a widely cited paper, McGinnis and Foege (1993) showed that unhealthy behaviors and environmental exposures were the "actual causes of death" that accounted for 50 percent of all U.S. mortality. Moreover, modern scientific tools afford far-reaching opportunities for unraveling mechanistic processes (e.g., environmentally induced gene expression, overload of physiological systems) through which behavioral and psychosocial factors contribute to illness and disease. In counterpoint to such maladaptive biobehavioral interactions, people's positive daily practices (e.g., getting proper nutrition, engaging in physical activity, avoiding cigarettes, alcohol, and drugs), along with the quality of their social relationships, psychological outlooks, and community supports are emerging as key ingredients to health and well-being over the life course. In short, the behavioral and social sciences are unavoidably implicated in making sense of both illness and good health, although much as yet is unknown about how these effects occur, particularly in terms of what can be done to avoid their deleterious impacts as well as promote their salubrious benefits for ever larger segments of the population.

This chapter sets the stage for the proposed new era of integrative health research. We first briefly review the history of the behavioral and social sciences at NIH and then describe the specific charge to the committee and our interpretation of this charge.

The integrative approach to health is the overarching theme of this report. In support of it, we revisit the distinguished intellectual history of those who have called for such bringing together of multiple levels of analysis. In numerous corners of science, the need to embark on new inquiries that put the disciplines together is a growing refrain. This synthesis—the move toward "consilience" (Wilson, 1998)—is particularly essential if we are to achieve comprehensive understanding of how good health at the level of the individual and of society is realized or lost. Much has been learned, and will continue to be gained, by focusing on single diseases and single mechanistic processes, but we bring into high relief the reality that many illnesses co-occur, as do many risk factors (behavioral and biological). What is needed, thus, are new studies that delineate the biopsychosocial pathways through which converging processes contribute to diverse health outcomes.

Each of the following chapters is broad and integrative in scope. Collectively, the chapters comprise key elements required for integration, from molecular, cellular, and genetic levels through behavioral, psychological, social, and environmental levels to multiple health outcomes. Stated otherwise, the chapters embody what the committee deemed critical influences that are essential to understanding the pathways to health.

THE CONTEXT: BEHAVIORAL AND SOCIAL SCIENCES AT THE NATIONAL INSTITUTES OF HEALTH

The behavioral and social sciences are increasingly recognized as vital contributors to understanding and improving the nation's health. In this regard, it is important to note the long history of behavioral and social science research at NIH. For example, the National Heart Institute, predecessor of the National Heart, Lung, and Blood Institute, was founded in 1948 and funded its first behavioral science research grant in 1955. The study was focused on psychological factors related to high blood pressure and coronary heart disease. The National Cancer Institute, established in 1937, also has an extensive behavioral research program emphasizing cancer prevention and control. The historical roots of this broad agenda reside in the mandate of the National Cancer Act, passed by Congress in 1971. More generally, many of the institutes have longstanding and well-developed behavioral and social science programs. Trans-institute initiatives with linkages to basic biology are also appearing with increasing frequency, such as the recent call for proposals on socioeconomic status and health as well as the recent establishment of five new mind/body centers around the country.

At the same time, the behavioral and social sciences have limited presence at some institutes or are seen as peripheral to primary agendas. Also, when considered at all, behavioral, psychological, and social priorities are sometimes restricted to a narrow focus on their role as risk factors for particular disease outcomes. To facilitate the growth and development of these important fields, Congress established the Office of Behavioral and Social Sciences Research (OBSSR) at NIH in 1995. A central message of OBSSR, and the background for this report, is that behavioral, psychosocial, and environmental factors have broad significance at NIH and are fundamental to comprehensive understanding of diverse disease etiologies as well as to positive health promotion.

THE CHARGE TO THE COMMITTEE

In 1999 the director of OBSSR requested assistance from the National Research Council (NRC) to develop a research plan to guide NIH in supporting areas of high priority in the social and behavioral sciences. Three principal goals shaped the OBSSR planning efforts: (1) enhancement of behavioral and social sciences research and training, (2) integration of biobehavioral interdisciplinary perspectives across NIH, and (3) improvement of communication between those conducting scientific research and the general public. The OBSSR sought to use the priorities requested from the NRC as a framework within which to implement these goals.

Within the NRC and its Commission on Behavioral and Social Sciences and Education (CBASSE), the Board on Behavioral, Cognitive, and Sensory Sciences chose to undertake a brief, highly focused study in response to the OBSSR request. The board established our committee to carry out this activity. Drawing on the existing social behavioral research base, the committee was asked to frame its discussion around four key areas:

1. behavioral and social risk and protective factors;
2. biological, behavioral, and social interactions as they affect health;
3. behavioral and social treatment and prevention approaches;
4. basic behavioral and social processes.

In addition, the committee was encouraged to consider the following issues in shaping its response: (a) health problems for which behavioral and social sciences research might offer solutions with respect to treatment and prevention, (b) areas of scientific opportunity in the behavioral and social sciences where a substantial investment might pay large dividends in the near future, (c) the public's chief health concerns.

Finally, the committee was asked to give special attention to collaborative research, interdisciplinary projects, and trans-institute initiatives that would have general application to broad areas of illness and health and would be sensitive to perspectives of the various NIH institutes. In considering this charge, the committee decided not to undertake a thorough review of all extant social behavioral research at NIH, a behemoth task beyond the scope of this report. Rather, guided by its original charge, the committee set itself to charting promising future directions where the behavioral and social sciences are well poised to connect with extant biomedical and/or intervention agendas (at individual, community, or population levels). Importantly, the members decided this could best be accomplished not by organizing the report around specific diseases or institutes, thereby following the current structure of NIH, but by providing a broader, more integrative approach.

It should be noted that the behavioral and social sciences, as applied to health, have never been organized around specific diseases. This is understandable, given that many behavioral risk factors (e.g., smoking, obesity, sedentary lifestyles, risky sexual practices) not only themselves co-occur but are also precursors to multiple physiological risk factors and multiple adverse health outcomes. The integrative approach thus gives much greater emphasis to the empirical realities of co-occurring risk and comorbidity, both of which are better understood with an integrative approach. The committee's essential task was to identify key components of a comprehensive approach as to how health outcomes, broadly defined, come about.

It is important to underscore three aspects of the committee's approach to its task. First, the committee covered a huge scientific territory in a very limited period of time and yet was able to quickly achieve consensus regarding the overall structure of the report and the content of the chapters. This efficient exchange was greatly facilitated by the prior experience of committee members in carrying out multidisciplinary science. There was little, if any, disciplinary turf guarding or vying for preeminence; instead, the targeted objective from the moment the work began was to find the best framework for integrating multiple fields and agendas.

Second, the committee had no intention of producing an exhaustive set of future research opportunities. Indeed, it is doubtful that such a comprehensive formulation could be developed by any committee. There was also no attempt made to cover extant programs of every institute within NIH. Stated otherwise, the committee was faced with the unavoidable requirement for selectivity. Nonetheless, the integrative research opportunities that it formulated do represent promising trans-institute initiatives, but they are put forth only as illustrations of the kinds of studies for which there could be substantial scientific payoff and opportunity to improve the public's health. Many vibrant areas of current NIH research are, therefore, inevitably missing from the chapters that follow. We state explicitly that what is not in the report is by no means an indirect message about low-priority status.

Third, the committee wrote this report with the scientific audience at NIH, and not the general public, in mind. Our goal is to communicate a new vision of integrative health to those who will carry out the future research and practice. A critical feature of such integration is the need to demonstrate command of complex areas and their interrelationships. Thus, we have not eliminated all technical details but tried to write about them so as to maximize their accessibility to our audience.

THE INTEGRATIVE APPROACH TO HEALTH

In the past 25 years, the study of human health has included a distinguished, but neglected, intellectual tradition put forth by numerous investigators, who saw the need for broad integrative frameworks that capture complex pathways to illness and disease. Engel (1977), for example, formulated a multifactorial model of illness, later subsumed under the rubric "biopsychosocial" that views illness as a result of interacting systems at cellular, tissue, organismic, interpersonal, and environmental levels. As a result, the study of every disease must include the individual, the body, and the surrounding environment as essential components. Lipowski (1977) and Fava and Sonino (2000) set the scope, mission, and methods of psychosomatic medicine as also involving interrelated facets of biological, psychological, and social determinants of health and disease. Around the same time, Henry and Stephens (1977) advanced a sociobiological approach to medicine and health that integrated not only biological, psychological, social, and physical environmental factors but also presented comparative studies of pathways to illness and disease between rodents, nonhuman primates, and humans.

More recently, Worthman (1999) combines human biology, life history theory, and epidemiology to consider variations in human development, giving particular emphasis to the role of hormones in the physiological architecture of the life course. Weiner (1998) offers "notes" toward a comprehensive evolutionary theory that integrates the roles of physical, social, environmental, and psychological factors in the maintenance of good health and the pathogenesis of disease. Keating and Hertzman (1999) assemble a cohesive set of essays that are designed to provide an "integration of knowledge about the determinants of health and human development." McEwen and Stellar (1993) introduce a multisystem approach to the cumulative physiological toll exacted by adverse behavioral, psychological, social, and environmental influences over the life course. This formulation of cumulative physiological risk is linked to unfolding interactions between genetic and environmental influences over time.

At an even broader level of thinking, E.O. Wilson has adapted and expanded on William Whewell's 1840 notion of consilience (Wilson, 1998, p. 8) as a "jumping together" of knowledge by the linking of facts and fact-based theory across disciplines to create a common groundwork of explanation. Wilson emphasized that "a unified system of knowledge is the surest means of identifying the still unexplored domains of reality. It provides a clear map of what is known, and it frames the most productive questions for future inquiry." Wilson's integration includes not only the full range of scientific disciplines but also the humanities and, as such, represents even more distant horizons for promoting health and well-being.

These perspectives collectively provide conceptual background to the theme of integration that guides this report and our related efforts to characterize pathways to multiple health outcomes. The time for this larger synthesis of scientific disciplines in pursuit of human health has come.

KEY INFLUENCES ON PATHWAYS TO HEALTH

Our task as a committee was one of identifying key elements that comprise an integrated and comprehensive approach to health. When the behavioral and social sciences are emphasized and linked to health, one is automatically led away from a disease-specific emphasis and into a view of multiple pathways to multiple outcomes. For example, smoking is a behavior linked to lung cancer, chronic bronchitis and emphysema, and cardiovascular diseases. Quality of social relationships, in turn, has been linked to cardiovascular diseases, later-life cognitive functioning, and recovery from a variety of illnesses. In both examples, and numerous others documented in this report, there is a need for understanding the pathways underlying these coarse-grained linkages. Moreover, full understanding of pathways requires a long time horizon that includes genetic predispositions and early life antecedents that contribute to later-life health and disease. It requires a multilevel view of life histories in which, for example, gene expression is seen as a dynamic process linked to psychosocial experience and community-level structures.

A behavioral and social science emphasis also leads naturally to a focus on prevention. This is not to detract from the social behavioral contributions to disease etiology, clinical medicine, and the organization and operation of the health care system. However, when the objective is to understand the mechanisms that explain how a range of health outcomes come about, it is appropriate and meaningful to identify health-promoting practices that can prevent or delay illness and disability and reduce the demand for curative health services.

With these observations in mind, the committee identified 10 priority areas for research investment that would integrate the behavioral, social, and biomedical sciences at NIH. These are briefly noted below, with emphasis on why they were selected and what they contribute to the larger mosaic of health.

Predisease Pathways: identification of early and long-term biological, behavioral, psychological, and social precursors to disease. This priority is intended to broaden the time horizons that guide research on disease etiology as well as underscore agendas that may lead to early preventive strategies.

Positive Health: identification of biological, behavioral, and psychosocial factors that contribute to resilience, disease resistance, and wellness. This priority draws attention to the need for greater emphasis throughout NIH on the biopsychosocial factors that help individuals maintain or regain good health throughout the life course.

Environmentally Induced Gene Expression: emphasis on the need to connect modern advances in genetic analysis to environmental factors (behavioral, psychological, social) to clarify their interactions in understanding positive and negative health outcomes.

Personal Ties: the growing body of literature that connects the social world to health and calls for greater explication of the biobehavioral mechanisms by which relationships with significant others (family, friends, coworkers) influence health and disease.

Collective Properties and Healthy Communities: greater emphasis on neighborhood and community-level variables, such as residential instability or social cohesion, and how they contribute to positive or negative health practices and outcomes.

Inequality and Health: builds in the growing awareness that socioeconomic hierarchies, racism, discrimination, and stigmatization are linked with differences in health and illness and calls for greater understanding of the mechanisms through which these effects occur and how they can be reversed.

Population Health: greater understanding of macro-level trends in health status, how the macroeconomy and population health are linked, and the performance of the health care system.

Interventions: expansion of the scope and effectiveness of behavioral, psychosocial, and biological strategies for improving health, including multilevel (individual, family, organizational, population) initiatives.

Methodology: emerges from the recognition that new measurement techniques and study designs are required to link information across diverse levels of analysis (molecular, cellular, behavioral, psychosocial, community) and across time.

Infrastructure: refers to the need for future structures and resources to maintain long-term study populations and train new generations of scientists to integrate health-related knowledge across multiple disciplines.

The scope of these priorities is expansive and integrative, with each encompassing wide areas of research. Some represent phenomena at the individual level, while others deal with macro-level (e.g. population) issues. The chapters that follow elaborate each of these priorities and identify principal recommendations associated with them. Collectively, they comprise the integrated pathway approach to health that is the guiding theme of this report.

REFERENCES

Engel GL. 1977 "The need for a new medical model: A challenge for biomedicine" *Science* 196:129-136.

Fava GA, Sonino N. 2000 "Psychosomatic medicine: Emerging trends and perspectives" *Psychotherapy and Psychosomatics* 60:184-197.

Henry JP, Stephens P. 1977 *Stress, Health and the Social Environment: A Sociobiologic Approach to Medicine* (New York: Springer-Verlag).

Keating DP, Hertzman C. 1999 *Developmental Health and the Wealth of Nations: Social, Biological, and Educational Dynamics* (New York: The Guilford Press).

Lipowski ZJ. 1977 Psychosomatic medicine in the seventies: An overview. *American Journal of Psychiatry* 134:233-244.

McEwen BS, Stellar E. 1993 "Stress and the Individual: Mechanisms leading to disease" *Archives of Internal Medicine* 153:2093-2101.

McGinnis JM, Foege WH. 1993 "Actual causes of death in the United States" *Journal of the American Medical Association* 270:2207-2212.

Weiner H. 1998 "Notes on an evolutionary medicine" *Psychosomatic Medicine* 60:510-520.

Wilson EO. 1998 *Consilience: The Unity of Knowledge* (New York: Alfred A. Knopf).

Worthman C. 1999 "Epidemiology of Human Development" Chapter 3, pp. 47-104, in Panter-Brick C, Worthman C (eds.). *Hormones, Health, and Behavior.* (Cambridge U.K.: Cambridge University Press).

2

Predisease Pathways

Research from animal and human studies has clarified that pathways to many disorders provide a basis for understanding and altering biobehavioral trajectories before disease is extant. One example is cardiovascular disease where a great deal has been revealed regarding the role of elevated cholesterol, homocysteine blood levels, hypertension, and abdominal fat, among other factors, in increasing risk for coronary atherosclerosis, stroke, and myocardial infarction. The detection of early warning signs with a high predictive value for later disease is an important aspect of prevention.

We use the term "predisease pathway" to describe the biological influences (e.g., genetic factors, endocrine and immune factors) and related links to behavioral, psychological, and social influences that precede morbidity and mortality. A primary message is the need to assess precursors to disease at points more distant temporally than has been examined in most previous research. Wider time horizons are required to understand early antecedents to later risk factors as well as the long-term etiological processes involved in multiple disease outcomes. Predisease pathways thus include a broad array of factors that affect the individual from conception (or before) through development and adulthood into later life. Illustrative influences include prenatal and early risk factors, along with a diverse array of psychological factors (e.g., control and efficacy, temperament, optimism, cognitive states, emotion regulation), behavioral factors (e.g., diet, exercise, smoking, alcohol consumption, drug abuse, sexual activity), and familial and environmental influences (e.g., social ties and support, family stress, work conditions, community supports).

Equally important is the need to integrate these biological, behavioral, psychological, and social precursors to disease. The importance of such long-term developmental integration has recently been underscored by Worthman (1999): "We do not have an integrated model of human developmental physiology that can assist us in thinking about how ontogenetic changes may mediate environmental effects on adult health outcomes." Emphasis on temporally distant and integrated assessment of psychological, social, and behavioral risk requires counterpart assessment of cumulative risk across multiple physiological systems, a topic that is addressed below.

CUMULATIVE PHYSIOLOGICAL RISK

Building on the guiding theme of integrative research (see Introduction), there is a need to assess physiological risk across multiple systems simultaneously. Illustrative of this objective is the broad framework of allostatic load (McEwen, 1998; McEwen and Stellar, 1993; McEwen and Seeman, 1999), which maintains that either repeated or continuous exposure to challenge or chronic underexposure and social isolation disrupts basic biological regulatory processes central to the maintenance of homeostasis and health. This model suggests that individuals (human or animal) exposed to challenge at vulnerable times (e.g., during early stages of pre- and postnatal development) or repeatedly during any period of life may experience overexposure to physiological responses that are outside normal operating ranges. Such overexposure comes about either because there are many challenges or because the turning on and turning off of the physiological responses is inefficient. This exacts a wear and tear termed "allostatic load." Factors that may increase allostatic load include genetic predispositions, adverse experiences from early development, poor health behaviors (e.g., diet, exercise, and substance abuse), and exposure to stressful environmental conditions across the life span.

Through repeated efforts to adapt to stressful circumstances, the organism experiences a cumulative multisystem physiological toll, leading to cascading, potentially irreversible interactions between genetic predispositions and environmental factors. Over time, these cascades can contribute to large individual differences in dysregulation of the hypothalamic-pituitary-adrenal (HPA) axis, impaired immune function, altered cardiovascular reactivity, and ultimately stress-related physical and mental disorders (including chronic hypertension, coronary heart disease, diabetes, hippocampal atrophy and associated cognitive dysfunction; see Seeman et al.,

1997; Seeman and Robins, 1994; McEwen, 1998; Dhabhar and McEwen, 1996; McEwen et al., 1997).

Emphasis on allostatic load is not meant to overshadow the importance of diverse avenues of ongoing research on single systems of physiological risk (e.g., syndrome X and cardiovascular disease, dysregulation of the HPA axis and cognitive impairment). However, to date, there has been insufficient attention given to co-occurring risk across multiple physiological systems as well as to more temporally distant assessments of such risk. Because of its dual emphasis on cumulative risk across multiple physiological systems and cumulation across time, the concept of allostatic load is a particularly promising contributor to integrative health research, the theme of this report. Growing evidence of life course trajectories of comorbidity (i.e., individuals are ever more likely to suffer from multiple chronic conditions as they age) further underscores the importance of attending to co-occurring risk factors and their cumulation through time. Specifically, 45 percent of women and 35 percent of men ages 60-69 report two or more chronic conditions; figures rise to 61 percent of women and 47 percent of men ages 70-79 and 70 percent of women and 53 percent of men ages 80-89 (Jaur and Stoddard, 1999). Understanding the etiology of these comorbid profiles requires attending to multiple co-occurring risk factors.

A provisional operationalization of allostatic load has been provided by Seeman et al. (1997, unpublished manuscript), using measures of the HPA axis (cortisol, dihydroepiandrosterone sulfate), sympathetic nervous system (epinephrine, norepinephrine), cardiovascular activity (systolic and diastolic blood pressure), metabolism and adipose tissue deposition (waist-hip ratio), glucose metabolism (glycosylated hemoglobin), and atherosclerotic risk (serum HDL and total cholesterol). Underscoring cross-system linkages, high allostatic load was found in the MacArthur Studies of Successful Aging to predict later life mortality, incident cardiovascular disease, and decline in cognitive and physical functioning. Looking to socioeconomic and psychosocial precursors, the same operationalization has been linked to cumulative economic and social relational adversity from childhood through age 59 in a 40-year longitudinal study (Wisconsin Longitudinal Study; Singer and Ryff, 1999). A slightly modified version of this operationalization of allostatic load has been associated with lower levels of education as well as greater hostility in the Normative Aging Study (Kubzansky et al., 1999). We underscore the provisional nature of the operationalization of allostatic load, and in Chapter 10 we discuss in detail the future research program needed to refine assessment of cumulative physiological risk. In Chapter 3 we also discuss the optimal functioning of these multiple physiological systems via the concept of allostasis.

CHARACTERIZING PREDISEASE PATHWAYS

In addition to indicators of allostatic load, markers of the existence of individual diseases are becoming better known, leading to expanded prospects for understanding predisease processes. Some of these prospects stem from genetic advances that enable researchers to focus on mechanisms of predisease in vulnerable populations (e.g., people with genetic risk for Huntington's disease or breast cancer). Other prospects come from expanding knowledge of the physiological mechanisms underlying disease and corresponding markers. For example, in the case of HIV infection, CD-4 T-cell counts and viral load are reliable indicators of asymptomatic infection progression. Consequently, studying factors that influence how quickly or slowly such indicators progress will lead to insights regarding disease processes, behavioral cofactors, and the dynamics of the infection trajectory.

Scientific advances such as these expand the window of time within which disease processes may be examined. They open investigations to studying interactions among genetic predispositions, prenatal and early life influences on health trajectories, behavioral factors (e.g., poor health habits), and social psychological states across the life span. Each of these are implicated in the early stages of single or multiple health disorders and point to protective factors that may delay the course of illness or potentially reverse these trajectories.

Prenatal and Early Life Risk Factors

Prenatal experience plays a critical role in interacting with the genome to shape brain development, and these epigenetic influences in intrauterine life confer a set of predispositions that act across the life span to affect vulnerability for many chronic diseases (see Chapter 4). Optimal prenatal environments produce beneficial effects and adverse environments produce deleterious effects on the developing brain. For example, third-trimester placental corticotropin-releasing hormone (CRH) predicts incidence of preterm birth and fetal growth restriction (Wadhwa et al., 1993). The concomitant HPA products (adrenocorticotropic hormone and beta-endorphins) may be related to dysregulation of the HPA axis in offspring and to fetal learning (Sandman et al., 1997).

Both animal and human studies document the important role that quality of caregiving and parenting behavior plays in the development of stress regulatory systems. Animal studies demonstrate that variations in maternal care permanently alter the expression of behavioral, endocrine, and cognitive responses to stress. For example, as adults the offspring of rat dams who provided more maternal care during their first 10 days of life showed reduced plasma adrenocorticotropic hormone and corticosterone responses to acute stress, increased hippocampal glucocorticoid receptor messenger RNA expression, enhanced glucocorticoid feedback sensitivity, and decreased levels of hypothalamic corticotropin-releasing hormone messenger RNA (Caldji et al., in press). In humans, children exposed to parenting characterized by conflict, aggression, and neglect show disruptions in stress-responsive biological regulatory systems (sympathetic-adrenomedullary, HPA), poor health behaviors, and poor skills for emotional and social regulation (Repetti et al., in press). Abusive and neglectful family environments not only enhance risk for disease, injury, and premature death among children, they also interact with temperament to affect a broad array of mental and physical health disorders in adolescence and adulthood, including propensity for violence, depression, and risk for certain chronic diseases, including ischemic heart disease, some cancers, liver disease, and chronic obstructive pulmonary disease, a progressive disease process most commonly resulting from smoking (e.g.; Felitti et al., 1998; Walker et al., 1999).

Other early system dysregulations also are implicated in predisease pathways to adverse outcomes. Serotonergic dysregulation has been tied to enhanced risk for depression, suicide, and aggression, among other adverse outcomes. For example, depressed abused children showed elevated prolactin responses to a serotonin challenge, and those responses were correlated with clinical ratings of aggressive behavior and family history of suicide attempt (Kaufman et al., 1998). Animal studies suggest an important role for maternal behavior in moderating risk for serotonergic dysregulation. Here genetic risk factors play a role. For example, the short form of the 5-HTT allele, a gene related to serotonin transporter efficiency, confers low serotonin reuptake efficiency in monkeys, whereas the long form of the allele is associated with normal serotonin reuptake efficiency (Suomi, 1997). Monkeys with the short 5-HTT allele who were raised by peers (a risk factor for reactive, impulsive temperament) showed lower concentrations of the primary central serotonin metabolite (5-HIAA) than did monkeys with the long allele. But for monkeys raised by their mothers, primary serotonin metabolite concentrations were identical for monkeys with either allele. This pattern clearly suggests a protective effect of maternal behavior on expression of genetic risk for serotonin dysfunction.

Additional evidence for the interaction between genetic expression and early experience is provided by a study that randomly assigned rhesus monkey neonates selectively bred for differences in temperamental reactivity to foster mothers who were either unusually nurturant or within the normal range of mothering behavior (Suomi, 1987). Infants whose pedigrees suggested normal reactivity exhibited the expected patterns of biobehavioral development, independent of the relative nurturance of the foster mother. In contrast, dramatic differences emerged for the genetically highly reactive infants. Highly reactive infants cross-fostered to normal mothers exhibited deficits in early exploration and exaggerated behavioral and physiological responses to minor environmental perturbations. In adulthood they tended to drop and remain low in the dominance hierarchy (Suomi, 1991). Highly reactive infants cross-fostered to exceptionally nurturant females, in contrast, appeared to be behaviorally precocious. They left their mothers earlier, explored the environment more, and displayed less behavioral disturbance during weaning than both control (low-reactive) infants reared by either type of foster mother or highly reactive infants cross-fostered to normal mothers. In addition, when permanently separated from their foster mother and moved into larger groups, the highly reactive animals cross-fostered to nurturant mothers became adept at recruiting and retaining other group members as allies, and most became high dominant.

These primate studies are significant not only because they suggest an important role of parenting for modifying expression of genetically based temperamental differences but because they tie serotonergic dysfunction directly to behavioral attributes similar to those found in human offspring from abusive families. Specifically, monkeys raised without their mother (i.e., raised with peers) have difficulty moderating behavioral responses to rough-and-tumble play with peers, sometimes escalating those bouts into full-blown aggressive exchanges. Rearing with peers is also associated with a deficit of certain forms of prosocial behavior, such as less grooming among females. Peer-raised adolescent monkeys also show certain propensities for substance abuse, for example, requiring larger doses of the anesthetic ketamine to reach a state of sedation, and consistently consuming more alcohol and developing a greater tolerance for alcohol, compared to mother-raised monkeys. This pattern is predicted by their central nervous system's serotonin turnover rates, and thus serotonin plays a key role in the normal regulation of these behaviors. In human studies, difficulty in moderating aggressive impulses, problems in developing and maintaining social relationships, and risk for substance abuse are among the outcomes most consistently seen in response to the family environment characteristics of hostility and conflict, deficient nurturing, and parental neglect (Repetti et al., in press).

The potential intergenerational transmission of these behavior patterns also warrants note. Monkeys raised by peers (rather than by their mothers) are significantly more likely to exhibit neglectful or abusive treatment of their own offspring (especially firstborns) compared with their mother-reared counterparts (Champoux et al., 1992; Suomi and Levine, 1998). Exposure to effective parenting reduces these behaviors in both animals (Suomi, 1987) and humans. For example, interventions that modify family interaction patterns have demonstrated improvements in the behavioral concomitants of these dysregulations, such as drug abuse (Schmidt et al., 1996; see also McLoyd, 1998).

The underlying environmental conditions that give rise to these risky developmental pathways are increasingly understood and, again, parallels between human and animal studies are evident. Human conditions reliably associated with conflictual and abusive parenting include low or deteriorating socioeconomic status (SES), marital strife, and exposure to chronic stress. Comparable effects are seen in animal studies of caregiving under conditions of scarcity and exposure to other chronic stressors. A compelling example are the investigations of macaque mother-infant dyads maintained under one of three foraging conditions: low foraging demand (LFD), where food was readily available; high foraging demand (HFD), where ample food was available but required long periods of searching; and variable foraging demand (VFD), a mixture of the two conditions on a schedule that did not allow for predictability (Rosenblum et al., 1994). Exposure to these conditions over a period of months had a significant influence on mother-infant interactions, with the VFD condition the most disruptive. Mother-infant conflict increased in the VFD condition and infants of mothers housed under these conditions were significantly more timid and fearful. These infants showed signs of depression commonly observed in maternally separated macaque infants. As adolescents the infants reared in the VFD conditions were more fearful and submissive and showed less social play.

More recent studies have demonstrated the effects of these conditions on the development of neurobiological systems that mediate the organisms' behavioral and endocrine/metabolic response to stress. As adults, monkeys reared under VFD conditions showed increased cerebrospinal fluid levels of corticotropin-releasing factor (CRF). Increased central CRF drive, which reflects increased activity of hypothalamic and extra-hypothalamic CRF systems, such as are found in the central nucleus of the amygdala, is consistent with the role of CRF in anxiety and depression, and this is exactly what was seen in adolescent VFD-reared animals. These findings provide a mechanism for the increased fearfulness observed in the VFD-reared animals, which may then be transmitted to a subsequent generation of offspring. In a recent study in humans (Heim et al., 2000b), women with a history of childhood abuse exhibited increased pituitary-adrenal and autonomic responses to stress in adulthood compared to controls. The findings suggest that early life stress results in persistent sensitization of the HPA axis to mild stress in adulthood, thereby contributing to vulnerability to psychopathological conditions.

The examples of predisease pathways that thus far are tied to interactions between genes and early environment concern primarily HPA, sympathetic-adrenal-medullary, and neurochemical functioning. Appropriately timed measurements of serum or salivary cortisol, serum catecholamines, CSF levels of CRF and serotonin and catecholamine metabolites all provide clues as to the state of neural function in predisease states, and other measures need to be developed. The above-mentioned findings are well-researched examples of what is likely to be a broad array of system dysregulations in response to such gene-environment interactions. Other such system dysregulations may include but are not confined to alterations in dopaminergic regulation in noradrenergic and excitatory amino acid regulation, in the benzodiazapine system, in parasympathetic responses to stress, in metabolic functioning, and in reproductive functioning.

The parallels between animal and human investigations and the degree to which plausible pathways have already been mapped in these kinds of investigations underscores the importance of continued investigations of early routes to later disease from a perspective that examines the interactions among genetic, developmental, behavioral, social, and biological regulatory systems. For a superb review of symbiotic studies on humans and animals that exhibit such parallels, see Henry and Stephens (1977). For a lucid and more contemporary discussion, see Sapolsky (1994).

Psychological States

Three decades of psychosocial research have identified psychological states that are also implicated in predisease pathways. Such states interact with physiological predispositions, environmental stressors, and individual behavior to influence vulnerability to a broad array of illnesses, the trajectories of those illnesses, and their potential amelioration. These states include a sense of personal control or self-efficacy; the ability to regulate emotional experience; the development of social competence; temperamental states, such as optimism and neuroticism; cognitive states, such as positive or negative expectations regarding health; emotional states, such as depression and anxiety; and coping strategies, such as active versus avoidant coping. We highlight here some specific examples of the importance of these states in predisease processes.

A sense of personal control or self-efficacy is tied to a broad array of health-related outcomes. Self-efficacy is critically implicated in people's abilities to initiate and maintain good health habits, including exercise, breast self-examination, smoking cessation, and control of alcohol consumption (see Taylor, 1999, for a review). Interventions with patients awaiting noxious medical procedures, such as endoscopic examinations, reveal that even minimal interventions designed to enhance feelings of control (such as instructions in swallowing or attentional focus) permit these procedures to proceed with fewer complications (Johnson and Leventhal, 1974). Experimental investigations with institutionalized elderly have found that control-enhancing manipulations (such as the ability to choose when to participate in activities or when to have visitors) are associated with improved health and longevity (Schulz, 1976; Langer and Rodin, 1976). One study found that rats implanted with a cancerous tumor preparation and exposed to inescapable electric shock were less likely to reject the tumor preparation than animals exposed to no shock or to escapable electric shock (Visintainer et al., 1983). Experiences of control or self-efficacy affect health outcomes across the life span and in manifold ways, ranging from initial vulnerability to adherence to treatment.

Emotion regulation is implicated in the early stages of health disorders, ties that have been most clearly demonstrated in investigations of anger and hostility. Hostility is a risk factor for coronary heart disease in adult men (Dembroski et al., 1985), and in women antagonistic hostility is related to high levels of low-density lipoprotein cholesterol, high levels of triglycerides, and a higher ratio of high-density lipoprotein cholesterol to total cholesterol (Suarez et al., 1998). Emotional suppression, a form of emotion regulation, reduced expressive behavior in adult men and women and produced a mixed physiological state characterized by decreased somatic activity and decreased heart rate, along with increased blinking and indications of increased sympathetic nervous system activity (Gross and Levenson, 1993).

The antecedents of emotion regulation are laid down in early childhood. A high frequency of negative interactions between parents and sons predicted the sons' later hostile attitudes and outward expressions of anger (Matthews et al., 1996). Children of hypertensive parents show elevated systolic blood pressure reactivity to angry exchanges between adults, which may be a precursor of later difficulties in stress management and risk for hypertension (Ballard et al., 1993). A large body of literature suggests that a genetic risk for heightened sympathetic-adrenal-medullary reactivity to stress is exacerbated by familial transmission of hypertension through repeated exposure to such hostile episodes, resulting in a hostile interpersonal style in adulthood (Ewart, 1991). The fact that hostility can be significantly modified in interventions for people diagnosed with coronary heart disease and the subsequent effects these interventions have on risk factors (Blumenthal et al., 1988) suggests the potential importance of modifying emotional regulation early.

Temperamental states such as optimism interact with physiological states to moderate predisease pathways. For example, optimism was associated with higher numbers of helper T cells and higher natural killer cell cytotoxicity in students undergoing the stress of first-year law school (Segerstrom et al., 1998). Because these immune changes can be precursors to significant clinical states, including depression, anxiety, and vulnerability to infectious disorders, these results suggest potentially protective effects of optimism on predisease processes. This is a topic warranting further research, since the immune system can exhibit considerable fluctuation (plasticity) while remaining within normal operating range. A pessimistic explanatory style, namely the tendency to explain negative events in terms of internal, stable, global qualities in oneself, may represent a general risk factor for disease and early mortality. In one study, pessimistic explanatory style was measured at age 25 and health at ages 45 to 60 (Peterson et al., 1988). Those high in pessimistic explanatory style had significantly poorer health two to three decades later. A study of elderly people showed that those with a pessimistic explanatory style had compromised cell-mediated immunity (Kamen-Siegel et al., 1991), which may represent elevated risk for immune-related disorders in this vulnerable population.

Negative affective states adversely affect vulnerability and the courses of a range of health disorders. For example, chronic negative affect was associated with more severe respiratory illness (measured as mucous production) following experimentally induced exposure to a cold virus (Cohen et al., 1995). A meta-analysis revealed an association between prior depression and subsequent development of coronary heart disease (Booth-Kewley and Friedman, 1987). Among already diagnosed patients, those who became depressed in response to their diagnosed coronary artery disease were more likely to have a more debilitating course of illness and a repeat cardiac event, after controlling for other risk factors (Frasure-Smith et al., 1995).

The broad base of empirical evidence demonstrating the significance of these and related psychological states in pathways to many acute and chronic disease outcomes underscores the importance of continuing to explore their role in initiating, exacerbating, and moderating these predisease processes.

Behavioral Factors

A set of behavioral risk factors, including poor diet, little exercise, promiscuous and/or unprotected sexual activity, smoking, alcohol abuse, and drug abuse, is associated with a broad array of diseases. Continued attention to the development and modification of these behaviors is essential.

Research suggests intergenerational transfer of risk behaviors that point to the necessity for early intervention. For example, mothers who smoked during pregnancy were more likely to have adolescent daughters who smoked, even after controlling for the mothers' postnatal smoking histories (Kandel et al., 1994); this suggests that nicotine or other substances in tobacco released by maternal smoking may have affected the fetus, perhaps through nicotinic input to the dopaminergic system. These changes appear to predispose the brain during a critical period of its development to the subsequent addictive influence of nicotine more than a decade later. Other forms of substance abuse, such as alcohol and addictive drugs, appear to have similar prenatal effects, altering gene expression to produce lasting functional and structural changes in the brain. For example, intergenerational transmission of susceptibility to morphine and cocaine addiction has been demonstrated in animal studies (Beitner-Johnston et al., 1992).

People who use any type of drug are likely to use others (Capaldi et al., 1996; Donovan and Jessor, 1985; Kandel and Yamaguchi, 1993), which suggests that the drugs may share common biological substrates and/or serve common functions. Specifically, there is evidence that substance abuse helps individuals cope with dysregulated serotonin by facilitating release and/or impeding reuptake of the neurotransmitter. Dysregulation of serotonin and of the dopamine system is also tied to adverse early environments in animal and human studies. A likely pathway to clusters of poor health habits, then, is suggested by genetic risk interacting with challenging prenatal or early childhood conditions to produce serotonergic dysregulation, which is then "treated" through multiple poor health habits (especially those involving addictive substances) that represent efforts at self-medication.

Prospects for modifying these behaviors have expanded in recent years. For example, "stage models" of behavior change provide important insights into the modification of risk factors for disease and the corresponding predisease pathways they implicate. When trying to change health behaviors, people go through a series of stages that influence their receptivity to different kinds of interventions. This observation laid the groundwork for matching the type of intervention to the stage of readiness to change. For example, individuals still considering whether to change a behavior (such as stopping smoking) are best approached through persuasive communications that highlight the benefits of change, whereas those already committed to change may be best served by interventions that induce them to make explicit commitments to change and that provide training for bridging the gap between intentions and action. Similarly, strategies of relapse prevention are best directed to those facing the problem of long-term maintenance. This matching approach has been successfully applied to smoking cessation, quitting cocaine, weight control, modification of a high-fat diet, adolescent delinquent behavior, practice of safe sex, condom use, sunscreen use, exercise, and obtaining regular mammograms (Prochaska, 1994; Prochaska et al., 1992).

A lesson learned from secondary prevention concerns modification of multiple behavioral risk factors simultaneously (such as diet, exercise, and stress management). The strategy is to identify effective ingredients from studies of single-risk-factor behavior change programs and combine them into packages of effective multibehavior change programs. For example, for people with insulin-dependent diabetes, multilevel programs aimed at the simultaneous problems of weight control, glucose management, diet control, exercise, and stress management have the strongest impact on disease course when they are put together in a package and the elements of each segment are linked to each other (Wing et al., 1986). Such findings have implications for understanding predisease pathways through the alteration of multiple health habits as well.

Even when effective intervention packages have been created in research settings, there may be a gap between scientific knowledge and clinical practice. Despite demonstrated efficacy of research therapies in treating a broad array of disorders in children, adolescents, and adults (e.g., depression, phobia, other anxiety disorders), factors demonstrated to be effective in research are often not incorporated into clinical practice, consequently producing far poorer outcomes (Weisz et al., 1995). What is needed is careful attention to the design and implementation of effective intervention packages, so that they can become the standard of care administered by primary care practitioners.

Environmental Stressors

The social environment is critically important in influencing when disease processes will be initiated and what their course will be across the life span. Over 100 investigations of social ties and social support are testimony to the vital role these processes play in predisease pathways, as well as for disease course and recovery processes (Seeman, 1996).

The positive effects of the social environment on predisease processes begins very early. For example, in a review of more than 200 investigations of the determinants of adverse birth outcomes, social support from the baby's father or, in the case of unmarried girls, from their family members predicted beneficial birth outcomes, especially higher birth weight. These direct effects were indirectly mediated by less use of health-compromising substances such as cigarettes, alcohol, and drugs; better prenatal care; and lower stress (Dunkel-Schetter et al., in press). These health behaviors are inversely linked to risk of spontaneous abortion, fetal growth restriction, preterm delivery, and cognitive and motor deficits in offspring (Ness et al., 1999; Abrams, 1994).

The beneficial effects of social ties in adolescence and adulthood also are manifold. For example, individuals with higher levels of social ties were better able to avoid illness in response to experimentally induced exposure to a virus (Cohen et al., 1997). Such investigations suggest a significant role for social ties in predisease processes, specifically by reducing initial vulnerability, although the exact physiological and immunological mechanisms remain to be demonstrated. Nonetheless, there is substantial potential for using such findings to develop effective support-based interventions for improving health across the life span.

The differential distribution of social resources across SES levels and by racial/ethnic groupings also merits additional study. So understudied and important are social processes to predisease and disease outcomes that we devote parts of three chapters to their consideration, one on personal social ties (see Chapter 5), one on the collective properties of health environments (see Chapter 6), and one on the health consequences of inequality (see Chapter 7).

Environmental stressors are known to have effects, often dramatic, across the life span. Chronic stress can precipitate insulin-dependent diabetes in animals with a genetic risk (Lehman et al., 1991), and in children stressful life events increase the symptoms of juvenile diabetes (Hagglof et al., 1991). Animals given a malignant tumor preparation and exposed to a chronic stressor (crowding) showed higher rates of malignant tumor development than those not exposed to stress (Amkraut and Solomon, 1977). Evidence like this implicates stress in predisease pathways and suggests the importance of both research designed to identify the specific mechanisms involved in these risks and the development of interventions to modify stressors that may precipitate risk conferred by genetic or behavioral vulnerability.

Adverse effects of chronic stress exposure can be seen as early as the prenatal environment. Maternal stress at 18 to 20 weeks' gestation has been found to significantly predict corticotropin-releasing hormone (CRH) at 28 to 30 weeks' gestation, even after controlling for CRH at 18 to 20 weeks (Hobel et al., 1999). Research on adult populations has identified potential early signs of disordered physiological functioning in populations undergoing intensely stressful events. Research on populations affected by Hurricane Andrew ties stress exposure to alterations in immune functioning, including reductions in natural killer cell cytotoxicity and numbers of CD-4 and CD-8 T cells (Ironson et al., 1997). There is, as yet, no clear evidence that these perturbations are linked to downstream health outcomes. This underscores, however, the importance of investigating the plasticity of the immune system and clarifying which immune system parameters should be included in future operationalizations of allostatic load. Post-traumatic stress disorder (PTSD) is associated in some studies with increased cortisol, epinephrine, norepinephrine, testosterone, and thyroxin functioning, changes that last over a long period of time (Wang and Mason, 1999). However, hypocortisolism has also been implicated in response to PTSD (Heim et al., 2000a; Thaller et al., 1999; Ehlert et al., 1999) and even for healthy individuals living under conditions of chronic stress (Heim et al., 2000b). Exposure to combat in war is tied to the development of deviant thyroid profiles. (Indeed, a history of traumatic stress is one of the most reliable factors predicting thyrotoxicosis.) These alterations in thyroid functioning in response to traumatic stress are detectable more than 50 years later and thus appear to represent permanent alterations in physiological regulation in response to these intense stressors (Wang and Mason, 1999). Knowledge of such changes provides bases for hypothesizing and testing predisease pathways that may be implicated in adverse long-term health outcomes.

The workplace is an important source of both adverse and protective health effects across the life span. Among the workplace stressors that threaten health are low control over work activities, high work demands, low rewards, and combinations of these factors (Karasek and Theorell, 1990). Workers exposed to high job strain (high demands, low control) showed higher levels of ambulatory blood pressure three years later; moreover, changes in job strain were associated with changes in ambulatory blood pressure (Schnall et al., 1994). These patterns suggest that job strain can be an occupational risk factor implicated in the etiology of essential hypertension. A longitudinal study of 10,308 civil servants designed to identify work-related predictors of mental and physical health found that the work characteristics of high effort/low reward and poor social relationships were associated with poorer physical, psychological, and social functioning five years later, after adjusting for potential confounding factors (Stansfeld et al., 1998). These same work factors are especially implicated in the likelihood that workers will develop cardiovascular disease (Schnall et al., 1994).

Unemployment is a profoundly important stressor associated with high rates of depression, anxiety, and self-reported physical illness. Active coping strategies, that is the ability to respond to unemployment with plans and activities designed to alter the situation, can offset these ill effects (Turner et al., 1991). Unstable employment and employment at multiple unrelated jobs were associated with premature mortality, and the predisease mechanisms that underlie these effects merit exploration (e.g., Pavalko et al., 1993; Rushing et al., 1992). Workplace investigations also identified protective factors implicated in health trajectories. For example, the ability to develop social ties at work, including ties with supervisors, act as protective factors against adverse health and mental health effects of work stress (Buunk and Verhoeven, 1991).

Changing patterns of combining work and family roles have been understudied for their effects on health, especially their roles in predisease pathways. These include the expanding role of work and corresponding diminishing leisure time among workers and how work can compromise the development of personal resources, such as stable marriages and families and other social ties that might otherwise contribute to the protection of health. The effects on women of combining family and work roles and the factors that influence whether and when these role combinations have adverse or beneficial effects on mental and physical health merits research attention (Repetti et al., 1989). For example, female caregivers for older demented adults experienced long-term changes in immunity and health as a result of combining this demanding role with existing home and work responsibilities (Kiecolt-Glaser et al., 1991). Nurses scoring higher on job demands had higher ambulatory blood pressure and heart rate during the workday and higher epinephrine in the evening, and married nurses had higher nighttime cortisol levels than did unmarried women (Goldstein et al., 1999). These findings suggest that both high work demands and a combination of job demands and role demands at home have identifiable potentially adverse effects on neuroendocrine and physiological profiles. These effects were stronger the longer these women had worked. For a superb discussion of women's work roles, their impact on mothers and their children and health consequences, all from an evolutionary perspective, see Hrdy (1999).

As these research examples attest, intensely stressful environmental conditions (e.g., the aftermath of a natural disaster, unemployment), geographic areas of intense chronic stress (such as crowded neighborhoods), and life domains in which intense change is occurring (e.g., changing patterns of combining work and family) present special opportunities to identify predisease pathways that, to date, have been understudied. These acutely and chronically stressful conditions create alterations in underlying physiology and neuroendocrine responses that may be precursors to adverse health and mental health conditions. Using such naturally occurring conditions and events as laboratories for investigating predisease pathways and identifying who is most at risk for adverse health effects can lead to substantial progress in understanding the parameters of predisease states, the mechanisms by which they develop, and subsequent progression to disease.

CONNECTING PREDISEASE PATHWAYS TO CUMULATIVE PHYSIOLOGICAL RISK

The preceding discussions of prenatal and early life risk factors, psychological states, behavioral factors, and environmental stressors address a wide array of precursors to illness and disease, focused largely on early life. As yet these diverse literatures have not been linked with cumulative physiological risk, as illustrated by the concept of allostatic load, in later life. Indeed, research on allostatic load has been conducted primarily in samples of adults and the aged. Thus, an important direction for future research on predisease pathways is to connect these diverse early life risks (biological, behavioral, psychological, environmental) to subsequent life course trajectories of allostatic load. It is, in fact, such early precursors that are believed to initiate the cumulative physiological wear and tear that the concept of allostatic load is intended to capture. Investigations along these lines will require increased assessment of co-occurring components of physiological risk (e.g., function of the cardiovascular system, the HPA axis, sympathetic nervous system function, metabolic risk, immune function) early in life as well as their long-term sequelae in later life comorbidity.

RECOMMENDATIONS

A basic research initiative throughout NIH should focus on predisease pathways. Such an initiative would, of necessity, emphasize the unfolding interactions between environmental influences and gene expression over time. It should include the following topics:

- identification of early markers of predisease states;
- examination of their genetic and environmental origins through animal and human studies;
- identification of behavioral risk factors in the exacerbation or amelioration of predisease pathways;
- prioritization of experimental and longitudinal research to chart these trajectories across the life span;
- focus on the mechanisms by which genetic influences, early life experiences, and behavioral and psychosocial risk factors across the life span interact, leading to accumulating physiological risk for a broad range of disease outcomes.

REFERENCES

Abrams B. 1994 "Maternal nutrition" in Cresy RK, Resnik R (eds.). *Maternal-Fetal Medicine: Principles and Practice, 3rd Ed.* (Philadelphia PA: WB Saunders) 162-170.

Amkraut A, Solomon GF. 1977 "From the symbolic stimulus to the pathophysiologic response: Immune mechanisms" in Lipowski ZJ, Lipsitt DR, Whybrow PC. (eds.). *Psychosomatic Medicine: Current Trends and Clinical Applications* (New York: Oxford University Press).

Ballard M, Cummings EM, Larkin K. 1993 "Emotional and cardiovascular responses to adults' angry behavior and to challenging tasks in children of hypertensive and normotensive parents" *Child Development* 64:500-515.

Beitner-Johnston D, Guitart X, Nestler EJ. 1992 "Neurofilament proteins and the mesolimic dopamine system: Common regulation by chronic morphine and chronic cocaine in the rat ventral tegmental area" *Journal of Neuroscience* 12:2165-2175.

Blumenthal JA, Emery CF, Walsh MA, Cox DR, Kuhn CM, Williams RB, Williams RS. 1988 "Exercise training in healthy type A middle-aged men: Effects of behavioral and cardiovascular responses" *Psychosomatic Medicine* 50:418-433.

Booth-Kewley S, Friedman HS. 1987 "Psychological predictors of heart disease: A quantitative review" *Psychological Bulletin* 101:343-362.

Buunk BP, Verhoeven K. 1991 "Companionship and support at work: A microanalysis of the stress-reducing features of social interaction" *Basic and Applied Social Psychology* 12:243-258.

Caldji C, Francis D, Liu D, Plotsky PM, Meaney MJ. In press "The role of early experience in the development of individual differences in behavioral and endocrine responses to stress" in McEwen BS, Steller E (eds.). *Handbook of Physiology: Coping with the Environment* (New York: Oxford University Press).

Capaldi DM, Crosby L, Stoolmiller M. 1996 "Predicting the timing of first sexual intercourse for at-risk adolescent males" *Child Development* 67:344-359.

Champoux M, Byrne E, Delizio R, Suomi SJ. 1992 "Motherless mothers revisited: Rhesus maternal behavior and rearing history" *Primates* 33:251-255.

Cohen S, Doyle WJ, Skoner DP, Fireman P, Gwaltney JM Jr, Newsom JT. 1995 "State and trait negative affect as predictors of objective and subjective symptoms of respiratory viral infections" *Journal of Personality and Social Psychology* 68:159-169.

Cohen S, Doyle WJ, Skoner DP, Rabin BS, Gwaltney JM Jr. 1997 "Social ties and susceptibility to the common cold" *Journal of the American Medical Association* 277:1940-1944.

Dembroski TM, MacDougall JM, Williams RB, Haney TL, Blumenthal JA. 1985 "Components of type A, hostility, and anger-in: Relationship to angiographic findings" *Psychosomatic Medicine* 47:219-233.

Dhabhar F, McEwen B. 1996 "Moderate stress enhances, and chronic stress suppresses, cell-mediated immunity in vivo" *Society for Neuroscience* 22:536.3 – p1350

Donovan JE, Jessor R. 1985 "Structure of problem behavior in adolescence and young adulthood" *Journal of Consulting and Clinical Psychology* 53:890-904.

Dunkel-Schetter C, Gurung RAR, Lobel M, Wadhwa PD. In press "Psychological, biological and social processes in pregnancy: Using a stress framework to study birth outcomes" in Baum A, Revenson T, Singer J (eds.). *Handbook of Health Psychology* (Hillsdale NJ: Lawrence Erlbaum).

Ehlert U, Wagner D, Heinrichs M, Heim C 1999 "Psychobiological aspects of posttraumatic stress disorder" *Nervenarzt* 70/9:773-779

Ewart CK. 1991 "Familial transmission of essential hypertension, genes, environments, and chronic anger" *Annals of Behavioral Medicine* 13:40-47.

Felitti VJ, Anda RF, Nordenberg D, Williamson DF, Spitz AM, Edwards V, Koss MP, Marks JS. 1998 "Relationship of childhood abuse and household dysfunction to many of the leading causes of death in adults" *American Journal of Preventive Medicine* 14:245-258.

Frasure-Smith N, Lesperance F, Talajic M. 1995 "The impact of negative emotions on prognosis following myocardial infarction: Is it more than depression?" *Health Psychology* 14:388-398.

Goldstein IB, Shapiro D, Chicz-DeMet A, Guthrie D. 1999 "Ambulatory blood pressure, heart rate, and neuroendocrine responses in women nurses during work and off work days" *Psychosomatic Medicine* 61:387-396.

Gross JJ, Levenson RW. 1993 "Emotional suppression: Physiology, self-report, and expressive behavior" *Journal of Personality and Social Psychology* 64/6:970-986.

Hagglof B, Bloom L, Dahlquist G, Lonnberg G, Sahlin B. 1991 "The Swedish childhood diabetes study: Indications of severe psychological stress as a risk factor for type I diabetes mellitus in childhood" *Diabetologia* 34:579-583.

Heim C, Ehlert U, Hellhammer D. 2000a "The potential role of hypocortisolism in the pathophysiology of stress-related bodily disorders" *Psychoneuroendocrinology* 25/1:1-35.

Heim C, Newport J, Heit S, Graham YP, Wilcox M, Bonsall R, Miller AH, Nemeroff CB. 2000b "Pituitary-adrenal and autonomic responses to stress in women after sexual and physical abuse in childhood" *Journal of the American Medical Association* 284:592-597.

Henry JP, Stephens P. 1977 *Stress, Health and the Social Environment: A Sociobiologic Approach to Medicine* (New York: Springer-Verlag).

Hobel CJ, Dunkel-Schetter C, Roesch SC, Castro LC, Arora CP. 1999 "Maternal plasma corticotropin-releasing hormone associated with stress at 20 weeks' gestation in pregnancies ending in preterm delivery" *American Journal of Obstetrics and Gynecology* 180/1:S257-S263.

Hrdy, SB. 1999 *Mother Nature: A History of Mothers, Infants, and Natural Selection* (New York: Pantheon Books).

Ironson G, Wynings C, Schneiderman N, Baum A, Rodriguez M, Greenwood D, Benight C, Antoni M, LaPerriere A, Huang H-S, Klimas N, Fletcher MA. 1997 "Post-traumatic stress symptoms, intrusive thoughts, loss, and immune function after Hurricane Andrew" *Psychosomatic Medicine* 59:128-141.

Jaur L, Stoddard S 1999. *Chartbook on Women and Disability in the U.S.* (Washington D.C.: U.S. National Institute on Disability and Rehabilitation Research).

Johnson JE, Leventhal H. 1974 "Effects of accurate expectations and behavioral instructions on reactions during a noxious medical examination" *Journal of Personality and Social Psychology* 29:710-718.

Kamen-Siegel L, Rodin J, Seligman MEP, Dwyer J. 1991 "Explanatory style and cell-mediated immunity in elderly men and women" *Health Psychology* 10:229-235.

Kandel D, Yamaguchi K. 1993 "From beer to crack: Developmental patterns of drug involvement" *American Journal of Public Health* 83:851-855.

Kandel DB, Wu P, Davies M. 1994 "Maternal smoking during pregnancy and smoking by adolescent daughters" *American Journal of Public Health* 84:1407-1413.

Karasek R, Theorell T. 1990 *Healthy Work: Stress, Productivity, and the Reconstruction of Working Life* (New York: Basic Books).

Kaufman J, Birmaher B, Perel J, Dahl RE, Stull S, Brent D, Trubnick L, al-Shabbout M, Ryan ND. 1998 "Serotonergic functioning in depressed abused children: Clinical and familial correlates" *Biological Psychiatry* 44:973-981.

Kiecolt-Glaser JK, Dura JR, Speicher CE, Trask OJ, Glaser R. 1991 "Spousal caregivers of dementia victims: Longitudinal changes in immunity and health" *Psychosomatic Medicine* 53:345-362.

Kubzansky L, Kawachi I, Sparrow D. 1999 "Socioeconomic status, hostility, and risk factor clustering in the normative aging study: Any help from the concept of allostatic load?" *Annals of Behavioral Medicine* 21/4:330-338.

Langer EJ, Rodin J. 1976 "The effects of choice and enhanced personal responsibility for the aged: A field experiment in an institutional setting" *Journal of Personality and Social Psychology* 34:191-198.

Lehman CD, Rodin J, McEwen B, Brinton R. 1991 "Impact of environmental stress on the expression of insulin-dependent diabetes mellitus" *Behavioral Neuroscience* 105:241-245.

Matthews KA, Woodall KL, Kenon K, Jacob T. 1996 "Negative family environment as a predictor of boys' future status on measures of hostile attitudes, interview behavior, and anger expression" *Health Psychology* 15:30-37.

McEwen BS. 1998 "Protective and damaging effects of stress mediators" *New England Journal of Medicine* 338:171-179.

McEwen B, Seeman T. 1999 "Protective and damaging effects of mediators of stress: Elaborating and testing the concepts of allostasis and allostatic load" in Adler N, Marmot M,

McEwen B, and Stewart J, (eds.). "Socioeconomic status and health in industrial nations" *Annals of the New York Academy of Sciences* 896:30-47.

McEwen BS, Stellar E. 1993 "Stress and the individual: Mechanisms leading to disease" *Archives of Internal Medicine* 153:2093-2101.

McEwen B, Biron CA, Brunson K, Bulloch K, Chambers W, Dhabar F, Goldfarb R, Kitson R, Miller A, Spencer R, Weiss J. 1997 "Neural-endocrine-immune interactions: The role of adrenocorticoids as modulators of immune function in health and disease" *Brain Research Review* 23:79-133.

McLoyd VC. 1998 "Socioeconomic disadvantage and child development" *American Psychologist* 53:185-204.

Ness RB, Grisso JA, Hirschinger N, Markovic N, Shaw LM, Day NL, Kline J. 1999 "Cocaine and tobacco use and the risk of spontaneous abortion" *New England Journal of Medicine* 340:333-339.

Pavalko EK, Elder GH Jr., Clipp EC. 1993 "Worklives and longevity: Insights from a life course perspective" *Journal of Health and Social Behavior* 34:363-380.

Peterson C, Seligman MEP, Vaillant GE. 1988 "Pessimistic explanatory style is a risk factor for physical illness: A thirty-five-year longitudinal study" *Journal of Personality and Social Psychology* 55:23-27.

Prochaska JO. 1994 "Strong and weak principles from progressing from precontemplation to action on the basis of 12 problem behaviors" *Health Psychology* 13:47-51.

Prochaska JO, DiClemente CC, Norcross JC. 1992 "In search of how people change: Applications to addictive behaviors" *American Psychologist* 47:1102-1114.

Repetti RL, Matthews KA, Waldron I. 1989 "Employment and women's health" *American Psychologist* 44:1394-1401.

Repetti RL, Taylor SE, Seeman TE. In press "Risky families: Family social environments and the mental and physical health of offspring" *Psychological Bulletin*.

Rosenblum L, Coplan J, Friedman S, Bassoff T, Gorman J, Andrews M. 1994 "Adverse early experiences affect noradrenergic and serotonergic functioning in adult primates" *Biological Psychiatry* 35:221-227.

Rushing B, Ritter C, Burton RP. 1992 "Race differences in the effects of multiple roles on health: Longitudinal evidence from a national sample of older men" *Journal of Health and Social Behavior* 33:126-139.

Sandman CA, Wadhwa PD, Chicz-DeMet A, Dunkel-Schetter C, Porto M. 1997 "Maternal stress, HPA activity, and fetal/infant outcome" *Annals of the New York Academy of Sciences* 814:266-275.

Sapolsky R. 1994 *Why Zebras Don't Get Ulcers: A Guide to Stress, Stress-Related Diseases, and Coping* (New York: WH Freeman).

Schmidt SE, Liddle HA, Dakof GA. 1996 "Changes in parenting practices and adolescent drug abuse during multidimensional family therapy" *Journal of Family Psychology* 10:12-27.

Schnall PL, Landisbergis PA, Baker D. 1994 "Job strain and cardiovascular disease" *Annual Review of Public Health* 15:381-411.

Schulz, R. 1976 "Effects of control and predictability on the physical and psychological well-being of the institutionalized aged" *Journal of Personality and Social Psychology* 33:563-573.

Seeman TE. 1996 "Social ties and health: The benefits of social integration" *Annals of Epidemiology* 6:442-451.

Seeman TE, Robbins RJ. 1994 "Aging and hypothalamic-pituitary-adrenal response to challenge in humans" *Endocrinology Review* 15:233-260.

Seeman TE, Singer B, Rowe JW, Horwitz R, McEwen BS. 1997 "The price of adaptation—Allostatic load and its health consequences: MacArthur studies of successful aging" *Archives of Internal Medicine* 157:2259-2268.

Seeman TE, Singer B, Rowe JW, McEwen BS. Unpublished manuscript "Allostatic load as a measure of cumulative physiological risk: Is it more than syndrome X?"

Segerstrom SC, Taylor SE, Kemeny ME, Fahey JL. 1998 "Optimism is associated with mood, coping, and immune change in response to stress" *Journal of Personality and Social Psychology* 74:1646-1655.

Singer B, Ryff CD 1999 "Hierarchies of life histories and associated health risks" in Adler N, Marmot M, McEwen B, and Stewart J (eds.). "Socioeconomic status and health in industrial nations" *Annals of the New York Academy of Sciences* 896:96-115.

Stansfeld SA, Bosma H, Hemmingway H, Marmot MG. 1998 "Psychosocial work characteristics and social support as predictors of S-36 health functioning: The Whitehall II study" *Psychosomatic Medicine* 60:247-255.

Suarez EC, Bates MP, Harralson TL. 1998 "The relation of hostility to lipids and lipoproteins in women: Evidence for the role of antagonistic hostility" *Annals of Behavioral Medicine* 20:59-63.

Suomi SJ. 1987 "Genetic and maternal contributions to individual differences in rhesus monkey biobehavioral development" in Krasnegor NA, Blass EM, Hofer MA, Smotherman WP (eds.). *Perinatal Development: A Psychobiological Perspective* (New York: Academic Press) 397-420.

Suomi SJ. 1991 "Up-tight and laid-back monkeys: Individual differences in the response to social challenges" in Brauth S, Hall W, Dooling R (eds.). *Plasticity of Development* (Cambridge MA: MIT Press) 27-56.

Suomi SJ. 1997 "Early determinants of behaviour: Evidence from primate studies" *British Medical Bulletin* 53:170-184.

Suomi SJ, Levine S. 1998 "Psychobiology of intergenerational effects of trauma: Evidence from animal studies" in Danieli Y (ed.). *Intergenerational Handbook of Multigenerational Legacies* (New York: Plenum Press) 623-637.

Taylor SE. 1999 *Health Psychology 4th Ed.* (Boston MA: McGraw-Hill).

Thaller, V, Vrkljan M, Hotujac L, Thakore J. 1999 "The potential role of hypocortisolism in the pathophysiology of PTSD and psoriasis." *Collegium Antropologicum* 23(2):611-619.

Turner JB, Kessler RC, House JS. 1991 "Factors facilitating adjustment to unemployment: Implications for intervention" *American Journal of Community Psychology* 19:521-542.

Visintainer MA, Seligman ME, Volpicelli JR. 1983 "Helplessness, chronic stress, and tumor development" *Psychosomatic Medicine* 45:17 (Abstract).

Wadhwa PD, Sandman CA, Porto M, Dunkel-Schetter C, Garite TJ. 1993 "The association between prenatal stress and infant birth weight and gestational age at birth: A prospective investigation" *American Journal of Obstetrics and Gynecology* 169/4:858-865.

Walker EA, Gelfand A, Katon WJ, Koss MP, Von Korff M, Bernstein D, Russo J. 1999 "Adult health status of women with histories of childhood abuse and neglect" *American Journal of Medicine* 107/4:332-339.

Wang S, Mason J. 1999 "Elevations of serum T3 levels and their associations with symptoms in World War II veterans with combat-related posttraumatic stress disorder: Replication of findings in Vietnam combat veterans" *Psychosomatic Medicine* 61:131-138.

Weisz JR, Donenberg GR, Han SS, Weiss B. 1995 "Bridging the gap between laboratory and clinic in child and adolescent psychotherapy" *Journal of Consulting and Clinical Psychology* 63:688-701.

Wing RR, Epstein LH, Nowalk MP, Lamparski DM. 1986 "Behavioral self-regulation in the treatment of patients with diabetes mellitus" *Psychological Bulletin* 99:78-89.

Worthman C. 1999 "Epidemiology of human development" in Panter-Brick C, Worthman C (eds.). *Hormones, Health, and Behavior.* (Cambridge U.K.: Cambridge University Press) 47-104.

3
Positive Health:
Resilience, Recovery, Primary
Prevention, and Health Promotion

The structure of the National Institutes of Health (NIH) reflects a central focus on illness and disease. Most of the institutes are organized around major health problems (alcohol abuse and alcoholism; allergy and infectious disease; arthritis, musculoskeletal, and skin diseases; cancer; drug abuse; deafness and communication disorders; diabetes and digestive and kidney diseases; cardiovascular, lung, and blood diseases; neurological disorders and stroke; retinal and corneal disease). Among institutes with a nonspecific disease purview (aging, child health and human development, environmental health sciences, genome research, mental health, nursing), the preponderant program emphasis has also been on illness, dysfunction, and disorder.

As a much-needed counterpoint to long-standing focus on illness and disease, we urge the NIH to invest significant new resources in advancing knowledge of positive health. Such a program builds on emerging studies of resilience and resistance to adverse health outcomes (e.g., Glantz and Johnson, 1999) as well as current work on recovery from illness (e.g., Berkman et al., 1992; Leedham et al., 1995) and primary prevention (e.g., Raczynski and DiClemente, 1999; National Advisory Mental Health Council, 1998). Going beyond efforts to resist disease or recover from it, the focus on positive health also encompasses the need to understand and promote optimal human functioning. This requires attending to how and why individuals thrive and flourish (Ickovics and Park, 1998; Ryff and Singer, 1998a), qualities that embody the essence of good health, a central mandate of NIH.

Across the spectrum of inquiry on resilience, recovery, prevention, and positive health promotion, we underscore the fundamental importance of behavioral, environmental, psychological, and social factors. Research implicates these factors in the pathogenesis of multiple disease outcomes. Thus, reducing profiles of risk associated with negative behavioral, environmental, and psychosocial influences must be a key target for avoiding adverse health outcomes or delaying their onset. The positive health focus, however, calls for more, namely, the promoting of positive behavioral, environmental, and psychosocial factors viewed as protective influences in "salutogenesis" (Antonovsky, 1987)—the etiology of optimal health and well-being. A key implication of the shift toward positive health promotion is that it will require going beyond strategies targeted at high-risk groups to broader goals of health enhancement for the population at large (Rose, 1992). In the latter context, the goal is to shift entire population distributions toward better health, not just to intervene with special groups showing high risk.

From a historical perspective, we underscore the limited attention given to promotion of positive health, as contrasted with efforts to prevent, treat, or alleviate negative health outcomes. Despite the long-standing imbalance, current studies document that those with psychosocial strengths show delayed onset of symptoms as well as extended survival (e.g., Taylor et al., 2000), and the underlying mechanisms for such findings are poorly understood. Critically needed are future investigations of the physiological mechanisms (pathways) through which positive behavioral and psychosocial factors promote health, well-being, and longevity.

The preceding chapter on predisease pathways describes cumulative physiological risk as illustrated by the concept of allostatic load. Focusing on positive biological mechanisms, the concept of allostasis captures the capacity of the organism to adapt over the life course to oncoming challenges, thereby preventing the unfolding of pathophysiological processes (McEwen and Stellar, 1993). Allostasis emphasizes that the internal milieu varies to meet perceived and anticipated demands. That is, systems like the hypothalamic-pituitary-adrenal (HPA) axis and the autonomic nervous system exhibit large variations that actually help maintain other homeostatic systems (e.g., pH, body temperature, oxygen tension). This maintenance of "stability through change" (i.e., allostasis) promotes adaptation and appears to be importantly linked to social and behavioral factors, although current knowledge must be greatly expanded to understand the scope of these effects and how they come about.

Going beyond effective management of challenge and stress, the focus on positive health also points to the promise and potential of salubrious biobehavioral linkages. For example, recent findings on exercise and plasticity of the brain show that physical activity in rats increases BDNF, a growth factor of the neurotrophin family supporting the function and survival of many neurons (Neeper et al., 1995). Exposure of adult mice to enriched environments also increases neurogenesis in the dentate gyrus (van Praag et al., 1999). This increased cell proliferation, however, involved voluntary running, not maze running or yoked swimming, thereby underscoring the fine-tuned nature of positive biobehavioral linkages.

We urge that the scope of a positive health program at NIH be broad and integrative, running from molecular and cellular levels of analysis through neurophysiological systems to behavioral, environmental, and psychosocial levels of analysis. This is a call for increased support for multidisciplinary investigations that are centrally concerned with bridging between biomedical and social behavioral research. These have frequently been studied as separate realms or, when put together, have typically focused on adverse health consequences of maladaptive behaviors or on psychosocial stress and dysfunction. Comprehensive biopsychosocial understanding of how illness and disease are prevented (or delayed), as well as how positive health is promoted, is an overdue and much-needed priority, and we strongly encourage NIH to launch a new trans-institute initiative under the broad umbrella of positive health.

RESILIENCE AND RESISTANCE TO DISEASE: WHO STAYS WELL AND WHY?

Across NIH, there is pervasive concern for risk factors (genetic, behavioral, environmental) that predict the onset of particular disease outcomes. Scientific attention has focused disproportionately on individuals who ultimately suffer adverse health outcomes and on the etiological routes through which such effects occur. While the importance of such programs goes undisputed, we stress the concomitant need for studies of people with known risk factors who do *not* develop the disorder or disease in question. This resistance is usefully illustrated with samples pertaining to genetic risk.

Among females with the $BRCA_1$ gene, about 29 percent develop ovarian cancer by age 50 and 50 percent by age 85 (Ford et al., 1995). More than half do not develop the disease, despite having genetic risk. Similarly, among those with the DYT_1 gene for idiopathic torsion dystonia, only about 30 percent develop the disease (Risch et al., 1995). The gene for familial dysautonomia (localized to chromosome 9Q31) is carried by 30 percent of Ashkenazi Jews, but the development of this hereditary sensory dysfunction is so sensitive to diverse environmental triggers (e.g., cumulative stress, persistent infections) that no single summary penetrance number is meaningful (Blumenfeld et al., 1993). Of those with genetic risk of primary pulmonary hypertension (25-27 region on chromosome 2q31-32), the frequency of developing the disease at some point in a lifetime is only

10-20 percent (Rich, 1998). Finally, the expression of Type 1 diabetes among those with genetic susceptibility (major histocompatibility complex on chromosome 6p21 and 17 *and* a 14/15 base pair oligonucleotide on chromosome 11p15) is very sensitive to diet, infections, and a range of external environmental triggers (Todd, 1999).

All of the above examples underscore the importance of understanding disease resistance or delay of onset in the face of high risk. Given the dominant focus on predicting disease incidence, rather than avoidance, such inquiry represents largely uncharted scientific territory. It is nonetheless essential for mapping the causal processes involved in disease resistance, particularly in the face of known risk. Behavioral and psychosocial factors (e.g., exercise, nutrition, coping strategies, optimism, social supports) are not necessarily implicated in all such instances. Other genetic factors, for example, may account for aspects of disease resistance, but even these routes need to be explicated, particularly with regard to the nature of environmentally induced gene expression.

Even the most powerful environmental risk factors do not produce uniform outcomes. In studies of children growing up under adverse environmental conditions (e.g., parental psychopathology, parental alcoholism, extreme poverty), some children exhibit remarkable resilience, as evidenced by profiles of healthy development and avoidance of the disorders that characterize their parents (Garmezy, 1991; Glanz and Johnson, 1999; Rutter, 1990; Werner and Smith, 1992). These individuals have "defied others' expectations and survived or surmounted daunting and seemingly overwhelming dangers, obstacles and problems" (Leshner, 1999). Numerous protective factors have been suggested to explain such resilience (e.g., having bonds with at least one nurturing and supportive parent, receiving support from the external community, having an affectionate and outgoing temperament). Intervention studies conducted with children of poverty or those with developmental disabilities also show that significant improvements in cognitive, academic, and social outcomes can be promoted among those lacking early resources or abilities (Ramey and Ramey, 1998).

A further realm for illustrating resilience pertains to the growing interest in social inequalities and health (Adler et al., 1999). A recent trans-institute initiative seeks to advance knowledge of how these effects occur by explicating the intervening behavioral, psychosocial, and neurobiological processes. Existing research shows that lower socioeconomic status (SES) increases risk for ill health, but there is extensive variability within SES groups. Not all individuals with limited life resources and opportunities have poor health; in fact, some show optimal physical and mental health. Greater scientific investment is needed to explain the behavioral, psychosocial, and biological protective factors that underlie class-related health resilience. For example, individuals with cumulative economic adversity are more likely to have high allostatic load, a predictor of later-life morbidity and mortality (Seeman et al., 1997). Those from deprived economic backgrounds who had offsetting benefits of good social relations (e.g., affectional ties with parents, intimacy with spouse) are significantly less likely to exhibit the physiological indicators associated with high allostatic load (Singer and Ryff, 1999). Additional studies are needed to identify protective factors among low SES individuals who defy the odds of succumbing to ill health.

Across the above examples, longitudinal studies are essential to ascertain whether observed resistance and resilience reflect higher starting baseline profiles or the influence of subsequent interventions and/or protective resources. Even more imperative is the need for investigations to establish the neurobiological mechanisms through which health protection occurs. While adverse outcomes, particularly under conditions of high risk, are avoided, it is unknown whether this reflects a reversal of neurophysiological systems, compensatory responses, or both. We underscore the potential of animal studies to advance understanding of these mechanistic questions and thereby offer critically needed complements to the above human research. For example, animals reared in emotionally impoverished environments react to stress more radically throughout their lives than those reared in enriched environments (Caldji et al., 1998). However, these effects are reversible; those exposed to inadequate nurturing in early life can, if subsequently reared by a high-licking and high-grooming foster mother, show normal functioning and healthy adult lives. Animal models add critically needed understanding of how such behavioral interventions regulate the development of neural systems.

RECOVERY AND DIFFERENTIAL SURVIVAL PROCESSES

Effective treatment of major health problems is a central priority across the NIH. Much existing work emphasizes differential survival rates as a function of various behavioral and pharmacological treatments. The positive health focus calls for increased inquiry across the specific disease foci on psychological, social, and behavioral factors that contribute to recovery from particular health problems and/or enhanced survival rates while living with disease. Advances in these directions are already underway, as shown by recent reports (e.g., *Behavioral Research in Cardiovascular, Lung, and Blood Health and Disease* by the National Heart, Lung, and Blood Institute (1998) and *Basic Behavioral Science Research for Mental Health* by the National Institute of Mental Health (1995). This report calls for further strides of this nature across the other institutes as well.

Numerous protective resources promote recovery processes and increase survival rates. At the psychological level, mounting evidence points to the importance of optimism and hope in the face of health challenge. Positive expectations have been shown to predict better health after heart transplantation (Leedham et al., 1995); optimists have also been documented to show quicker recovery from coronary bypass surgery and have less severe anginal pain than pessimists (Fitzgerald et al., 1993). In men who are HIV-positive, optimism has been shown to predict disease course and mortality. Such men who were asymptomatic and did not have negative expectations showed less likelihood of symptom development during the follow-up period (Reed et al., 1994). Importantly, HIV-positive men with unrealistically optimistic beliefs about their own survival actually lived longer (Reed et al., 1994). Those who were able to find meaning in their loss of a close partner maintained CD-4 T helper cells over the follow-up period and were less likely to die (Bower et al., 1998). Thus, optimism and meaning are resources that may preserve not only mental but also physical health (Scheier and Carver, 1992; Taylor et al., 2000). On the other hand, unrealistic optimism in specific situations may encourage actions that create unwanted risks of injury and disease (e.g., Avis et al., 1989; Svenson, 1978; Weinstein, 1998), and these possibilities must also be part of future agendas.

Other factors contributing to differential survival profiles include social and emotional support. Group psychotherapy programs that promote social support and emotional expression among women with breast cancer show multiple effects: reductions in anxiety and depression as well as increased survival time and lower rates of recurrence (Spiegel et al., 1998; Spiegel and Kimerling, in press). Survival after myocardial infarction also has been significantly associated with emotional support, even after controlling for severity of disease, comorbidity, and functional status (Berkman et al., 1992). The negative role of emotional factors in survival processes has been demonstrated with anger in the context of coronary heart disease (Kawachi et al., 1996) and depression among postmyocardial infarction patients (Frasure-Smith et al., 1993). Future studies are needed to document the replicability and pervasiveness of these effects.

Recent research shows that promoting the positive can help prevent relapse of depression, a central challenge for clinicians involved in the treatment of this disorder (Fava et al., 1998; Fava, 1999). This is particularly relevant to the residual phase of depression, when major debilitating symptoms have subsided but well-being is not fully regained. During this period the risk for relapse is especially high. To promote full recovery, "well-being therapy" was implemented—a cognitive behavioral approach designed to increase awareness of and participation in positive aspects of daily life. Those participating in treatment showed dramatically higher remission profiles over a two-year period compared to those receiving standard clinical treatment. This underscores the need to promote positive psychosocial and emotional experience as a key route to sustained recovery from depression.

Finally, relevant to the challenge of living with chronic disease, we call for additional emphasis on quality of life. Current approaches accentuate basic mobility and self-care capacities, along with effective management of treatment side effects (e.g., with medications for lowering cholesterol or blood pressure). In addition to clinical management of disease, a positive health approach would also include higher levels of functioning and well-being (e.g., self-esteem, efficacy and mastery, quality ties to others, purpose in life). Current psychosocial assessment tools have much to offer regarding enrichment of quality of life indicators and thereby to studies of health-related quality of life on survival. We endorse the report of the National Heart, Lung, and Blood Institute (1998, p. 19), which states that "health-related quality of life is a relatively new area of behavioral research. Nevertheless, it is likely to assume growing importance as the medical community and public increasingly recognize that patient's abilities to participate in life's major activities are an essential component of medical evaluation and decision-making." Of critical research significance, however, is whether enriched quality of life slows disease progression and thereby delays mortality. These are important targets for future inquiry.

ADVANCING THE SCIENCE OF PRIMARY PREVENTION

The concern of positive health extends beyond efforts to increase survival vis-à-vis disease; it also includes efforts to reduce the likelihood of adverse health outcomes via primary prevention. Compared to curative approaches, preventive medicine has received notably little attention (Rose, 1992). Prevention is not a science with a confirmed tradition (Raczynski and DiClemente, 1999, pp. 3-11) but rather a newly emerging, multidisciplinary field of inquiry involving the behavioral and social sciences as well as public health, medical, and other allied disciplines. We strongly endorse the need to advance the science of primary prevention, that is, the knowledge base on which prevention programs are built.

As a model for expanding preventive programs across the institutes of NIH, we draw attention to a recent National Advisory Mental Health Council report entitled *Priorities for Prevention Research at the NIMH* (1998). The report discussed basic biological, psychological, and sociocultural factors (and their interactive influences) involved in preventing mental disorders as well as relapse, comorbidity, disability, and adverse family consequences of severe mental illness. Among the core scientific recommendations were the needs to strengthen the epidemiological foundations of prevention research, stimulate early intervention studies in childhood, broaden the populations targeted for prevention research, support long-term follow-up in prevention studies, and build prevention research capacities through training grants. These priorities provide much-needed direction across other institutes as well.

Scientifically, prevention research has been overwhelmingly focused on the need to change behavior, specifically maladaptive behaviors that increase risk for disease. Extensive work has examined changing behaviors related to tobacco use (Winders et al., 1999), obesity and nutrition (Spear and Reinold, 1999), physical activity (Sanderson and Taylor, 1999), and alcohol and drug abuse (Schumacher and Milby, 1999). Behavioral changes needed to prevent specific health outcomes, such as cardiovascular disease (Raczynski et al., 1999), cancer (Reynolds et al., 1999), pulmonary disorders (Kohler et al., 1999), and HIV/AIDS (DiClemente et al., 1999) have also been studied. Prevention research has encompassed the life span (Albee and Gulotta, 1997; Millstein et al., 1993), including early interventions for children at risk, fostering resilient outcomes in children of divorce, promoting life skills training for adolescents at risk, and developing adult programs to promote reemployment following job loss.

These prevention endeavors bring to the fore issues of responsibility—that is, does the individual or the collective bear responsibility for enacting effective behavior change (Fischhoff, 1992)? Depending on the response, some programs have focused competence promotion and education at the individual level, including helping individuals make effective choices regarding their own health and well-being (Clemen, 1991; Dawes, 1988; Fischhoff et al., 1997), while others have addressed broader issues of environmental support and community organization (Albee and Gullotta, 1997). Prevention is thus a formidable challenge of wide scope, influenced not just by virus, gene, and physiological processes but also by individuals' cognitions, emotions, and behaviors, all of which exist within particular environmental, interpersonal, economic, and cultural contexts. Clearly, advancing the science of primary prevention is a multidisciplinary task.

The committee recommends that NIH usher in a new era of prevention research, spanning all institutes and targeted at a refined understanding of these complex connections. For example, adverse health consequences follow from numerous behavioral and psychosocial factors (problem drinking, smoking, sedentary lifestyles, poor stress management), and yet notably limited progress has been made in understanding why only one in four Americans exercises regularly or why the prevalence of smoking (especially among teenagers) remains unacceptably high (National Heart, Lung, and Blood Institute, 1998). Much prior work rested on the belief that informed individuals would make good behavioral choices: teach people about the dangers of smoking and they will not smoke; teach people about the danger of drugs and they will not use them; teach people about the importance of exercise and nutrition, and they will stay fit and eat properly. Unfortunately the relationships between information, education, and prevention are not clear-cut or direct (Rothman and Kiviniemi, 1999).

With regard to the science of primary prevention, it is also important to recognize the role of individuals as active agents, shaping their environment, evaluating the appropriateness of public policies and medical recommendations, following or abandoning therapeutic protocols, self-medicating with over-the-counter drugs, and so on. The effectiveness of programs designed to reduce health-risk behaviors or increase health-promoting behaviors depends on the interplay of individuals' beliefs, values, affective responses, and social interactions (Fischhoff, 1999; Merz et al., 1993). The creation of the NIH Council of Public Representatives reflects a commitment to improve interactions between the individuals' decisions and advances in biomedical research (Institute of Medicine, 1998). These activities should be encouraged and extended.

For example, at the same time that basic science is documenting the life-extending benefits of caloric restriction (Weindruch, 1996) and clarifying the genetic mechanisms through which these effects occur (Lee et al., 1999), there is an epidemic of obesity (Mokdad et al., 1999). The prevalence of obesity in the general population increased from 12.0 percent in 1991 to 17.9 percent in 1998, an increase observed in all states and both sexes. By the most stringent definition, more than half of U.S. adults aged 20 and over are considered overweight and nearly one-quarter are clinically obese (Wickelgren, 1998). While the experts may disagree as to whether the central health threat is increase in body fat per se or lack of physical activity, there is no disagreement that major behavioral and environmental change is needed to correct this increase in obesity (Hill and Peters, 1998; Taubes, 1998), estimated to cost more than $70 billion annually in direct and indirect health care costs (Wickelgren, 1998). Understanding how to redirect individuals' investment in diet interventions that have little chance of success or that increase health risks is part of this agenda. Comparative cost-benefit analyses of prevention- versus treatment-oriented approaches, across multiple health problems, also constitutes an important future research direction.

Cast more broadly, the etiology and persistence of health-compromising behaviors together should become a key research priority at NIH. Far greater attention must be given to factors such as the personal motivation, values, skills, and intellectual resources needed to change behavior and to whether surrounding contexts and environments support the needed behavioral change. These issues call for a new era of scientific studies of why maladaptive behaviors are so intransigent, particularly when knowledge of related health risks is widely available, and what can be done to modify these behaviors. Like our science, individuals may need a better understanding of health-promoting processes in addition to those associated with risk (National Research Council, 1989; Woloshin and Schwartz, 1999). Thus, increased dissemination to the larger public of effective prevention strategies must be a key NIH priority.

NEW DIRECTIONS IN POSITIVE HEALTH PROMOTION

While primary prevention is the cornerstone of good public health, the most proactive version of positive health is the promotion of optimal health behaviors and sustaining supportive environments. The distinction between primary prevention and positive health promotion is usefully illustrated with an intervention program designed to teach "life skills" to high-risk adolescents (Danish, 1997). This project rests on the observation that "to be successful in life, it is not enough to know what to avoid; one must also know how to succeed. For this reason, our focus is on teaching youth 'what to say yes to' as opposed to 'just say no'" (p. 292). The Going for the Goal (GOAL) program views early adolescence as an appropriate time to teach life skills, promotes interventions that simultaneously increase health-enhancing behaviors and decrease health-compromising behaviors, recognizes that those who do not have positive future expectations are at risk for engaging in health-compromising behaviors, and realizes that teaching skills is a critical route to changing behavior and cognition. Using a peer-teaching model, high school-aged adolescents teach life skills to both older and younger peers, emphasizing how to formulate and pursue positive life goals, including learning how to surmount obstacles to goal attainment. Since 1992, GOAL has been implemented in many cities. Students participating in the program achieve more of the goals they set, have better school attendance, and report fewer health-compromising behaviors (e.g., getting drunk, smoking cigarettes, violence) compared with those in control groups.

In addition to positive health promotion via life skills training, we reiterate the health significance of optimism and hope as well as of social and emotional support. While these are relatively new areas of inquiry, emerging evidence shows that such factors promote longer-term survival for those suffering from specific health challenges (see above), and these effects may be of even wider significance for the general population. Optimists and adults with low anxiety have lower ambulatory blood pressure and more positive moods than pessimistic and anxious adults (Räukkönen et al., 1999). Individuals growing up with feelings of warmth and closeness with parents had, 35 years later, decreased incidence of diagnosed diseases in midlife (coronary artery disease, hypertension, duodenal ulcers, alcoholism; Russek and Schwartz, 1997). Other recent advances in the social and behavioral sciences, such as studies of emotion coaching in parents (Gottman et al., 1996), positive emotions (Fredrickson, 1998), purpose and meaning (Wong and Fry, 1998), coping and problem solving (Thoits, 1994), thriving and flourishing (Ickovics and Park, 1998; Ryff and Singer, 1998a,b), represent diverse topics ripe for connection with biomedical studies, where their health-promoting effects can be fully investigated.

Perhaps the most extensive documentation of salubrious effects following from the social realm pertains to social relationships/social support and health. Epidemiological studies have mapped contributions of the social ties and integration to host resistance, reduced morbidity, and delayed mortality (Berkman, 1995; Cassel, 1976; House et al., 1988). Subsequent experimental studies and interventions have elaborated the beneficial effects of quality social interaction (e.g., Cohen et al., 1997; Spiegel, 1993). More recently, health behaviors and outcomes have been linked to religion and spirituality (Ellison and Levin, 1998; Koenig et al., 1998). Responsive to these findings, the National Institute on Aging has put forth a new program initiative on the connections between religion, spirituality, and health. Five newly funded centers for mind/body interactions will also carry forward the science of optimal health-promoting linkages between psychological factors and biology.

Some evidence exists that there are already trends toward positive health in some segments of the population. For example, recent population-level studies of the elderly show declining rates of disability among current cohorts of aged individuals (Manton et al., 1997; Singer and Manton, 1998). Even among older persons showing high disease burden, it has been shown that many do not become disabled (Guralnik et al., 1993). Other scientific research documents the capacities of many older persons to maintain or regain health status and functional capacities in the face of later-life challenges (LaCroix et al., 1993; Ryff et al., 1998; Staudinger et al., 1995). Thus, an emergent literature documents the growing prevalence of resilience in later life; however, the current work does not clarify the factors (behavioral, psychosocial, environmental, genetic) that contribute to the maintenance of functional capacities, health, and well-being in old age.

Critically needed across all these topics are entire new programs of research on the neurobiological mechanisms underlying the health benefits ensuing from behavioral and psychosocial influences. What are the actual processes (e.g., neural circuitry, endocrine and immune function) through which behavioral (e.g., nutrition, exercise, stress management) and psychosocial (optimism, purpose, coping, quality social ties) factors convey their health-promoting effects? This is a call to advance what is known about the "physiological substrates of flourishing" (Ryff and Singer, 1998a,b). Such inquiry has begun, for example, in studies linking social supports to physiological processes (Seeman, 1996; Uchino et al., 1996). These efforts have tended, however, to focus on the endocrinological and immunological correlates of relational conflict, or caregiving demands (Kiecolt-Glaser et al., 1996, 1997), not relational strengths. Thus, there is major need for new studies linking the positive aspects of social relationships (attachment, affection, intimacy) to the mechanisms that underlie good health (Ryff and Singer, 2000). Animal research provides valuable models for such explication of the mechanisms that connect positive social relations to health (Carter, 1998; Uvnäs-Moberg, 1997, 1998).

In sum, we urge NIH to embark on new programs of positive health promotion that will dramatically expand the scope of the above inquiries as well as related initiatives linking various behavioral (e.g., exercise, nutrition) and psychosocial (e.g., hope, meaning, support) to neurogenesis (Gould et al., 1997), anabolic systems and growth factors (Epel et al., 1998), and gene expression (Lee et al., 1999). The potential long-term payoff of early benefits following from these factors is critically important. That is, accompanying this call for greater emphasis on predisease pathways is a parallel need to advance knowledge of pathways of health promotion. Longitudinal studies are imperative to achieve this end.

POSITIVE HEALTH AND THE COUNCIL OF PUBLIC REPRESENTATIVES

The core objectives of the positive health focus are directly responsive to the input provided by the Council of Public Representatives (COPR), which brings public views to NIH activities, programs, and decisions (see Executive Summary). The strong message from COPR, speaking for the general public, was that NIH should do more to help people create and lead healthy lives. Many perceive NIH as focused on curing disease rather than on promoting quality living, optimal families, supportive work environments, and healthy communities. They also called for more information about how the general public can take more responsibility for its own health care. The behavioral and psychosocial research initiatives described under positive health are very much in the spirit of these messages from the general public. We have outlined multiple new directions at NIH for promoting optimal health via positive health behaviors (nutrition, exercise, stress management), quality social relationships, and strong psychological resources. These are core domains of ever-expanding knowledge in the social and behavioral sciences, but there is great need for linking them to ongoing biomedical programs across the institutes. The integration of these realms with an explicit focus on primary prevention and positive health promotion is a key route to improving the health of the U.S. population.

RECOMMENDATIONS

We urge NIH to promote new trans-institute programs to clarify the role of behavioral, environmental, and psychosocial factors in promoting optimal health. Such work should be targeted toward the general population and not focused solely on at-risk groups. Specifically, we recommend that NIH:

- target new research on the neurobiological mechanisms (e.g., allostasis, neurogenesis, anabolic systems, and growth factors) through which positive behavioral and psychosocial factors (e.g., exercise, enriched environments, quality social relationships, psychological well-being) influence health;
- establish new priorities focused on the etiology (at genetic, behavioral, and environmental levels) of disease resistance, particularly in the contexts of known risk;
- increase support for the study of protective resources (optimism, meaning and purpose, social and emotional support, and related neurobiological mechanisms) that promote recovery and increased survival rates;
- initiate new investigations that will advance knowledge of resilience in the face of life adversity, giving particular emphasis to longitudinal studies;
- advance the science of primary prevention, giving particular attention to overcoming persistent maladaptive behaviors (e.g., drinking, smoking, sedentary lifestyles, poor stress management);
- develop new population-based initiatives, implemented at local community levels, that promote health via the teaching of positive life practices and the provision of environmental supports to sustain them.

REFERENCES

Adler NE, Marmot M, McEwen BS, Stewart J. 1999 "Socioeconomic status and health in industrialized nations: Social, psychological, and biological pathways" *Annals of the New York Academy of Sciences*, 896, entire issue.

Albee GW, Gullotta TP. 1997 *Primary Prevention Works* (Thousand Oaks CA: Sage Publications).

Antonovsky A. 1987 *Unraveling the Mysteries of Health: How People Manage Stress and Stay Well* (San Francisco CA: Jossey-Bass Publishers).

Avis NE, Smith KW, McKinlay JB. 1989 "Accuracy of perceptions of heart attack risk" *American Journal of Public Health* 79:1608-1612.

Berkman LF. 1995 "The role of social relations in health promotion" *Psychosomatic Medicine* 57:245-254.

Berkman LF, Leo-Summers L, Horwitz RI. 1992 "Emotional support and survival after myocardial infarction" *Annals of Internal Medicine* 117:1003-1009.

Blumenfeld A, Slaugenhaupt SA, Axelrod FB, Lucente DE, Maayan C, Leibert CB, Ozelius L, Trofatter JA, Haines JL, Breakfield XO, Gusella JF. 1993 "Localization of the gene for familial dysautonomia on chromosome 9 and definition of DNA markers for genetic diagnosis" *Nature Genetics* 4:160-164.

Bower JE, Kemeny ME, Taylor SE, Fahey JL. 1998 "Cognitive processing, discovery of meaning, CD4 decline, and AIDS-related mortality among bereaved HIV seropositive men"
Journal of Consulting and Clinical Psychology 66:979-986.

Caldji C, Tannenbaum B, Sharma S, Francis D, Plotsky P, Meaney M. 1998 "Maternal care
during infancy regulates the development of neural systems mediating the expression of
fearfulness in the rat" *Proceedings of the National Academy of Sciences of the United
States of America* 95:5335-5340.

Carter CS. 1998 "Neuroendocrine perspectives on social attachment and love" *Psychoneuroendocrinology* 23:779-818.

Cassel J. 1976 "The contribution of the social environment to host resistance" *American
Journal of Epidemiology* 104:107-123.

Clemen RT. 1991 *Making Hard Decisions* (Boston: PWS-Kent).

Cohen S, Doyle WJ, Skoner DP, Rabin BS, Gwaltney JM Jr. 1997 "Social ties and susceptibility to the common cold" *Journal of the American Medical Association* 227:1940-1944.

Danish SJ. 1997 "Going for the Goal: A life skills program for adolescents" in Albee GW,
Gullotta TP (eds.). *Primary Prevention Works. Issues in Chidlren's and Families' Lives*,
Vol. 6 (Thousand Oaks CA: Sage Publications) 291-312.

Dawes RM. 1988 *Rational Choice in an Uncertain World* (San Diego CA: Harcourt Brace
and Jovanovich).

DiClemente RJ, Raczynski JM. 1999 "The importance of health promotion and disease prevention" in Raczynski JM, DiClemente RJ (eds.). *Handbook of Health Promotion and
Disease Prevention* (New York: Klewer Academic/Plenum Publishers) 3-11.

DiClemente RJ, Wingood GM, Vermund SH, Stewart KE. 1999 "Prevention of HIV/AIDS" in
Raczynski JM, DiClemente RJ (eds.). *Handbook of Health Promotion and Disease Prevention* (New York: Kluwer Academic/Plenum Publishers) 371-396.

Ellison CG, Levin JS. 1998 "The religion-health connection: Evidence, theory, and future
directions" *Health Education and Behavior* 25:700-720.

Epel ES, McEwen BS, Ickovics JR. 1998 "Embodying psychological thriving: Physical thriving in response to stress" *Journal of Social Issues* 54:301-322.

Fava GA. 1999 "Well-being therapy: Conceptual and technical issues" *Psychotherapy and
Psychosomatics* 68:171-179.

Fava GA, Rafanelli C, Grandi S, Conti S, Belluardo P. 1998 "Prevention of recurrent depression with cognitive behavioral therapy" *Archives of General Psychiatry* 55:816-821.

Fischhoff B. 1992 "Giving advice: Decision theory perspectives on sexual assault" *American
Psychologist* 47:577-588.

Fischhoff B. 1999 "Why (cancer) risk communication can be hard" *Journal of the National
Cancer Institute Monographs* 25:1-7.

Fischhoff B, Bostrom A, Quadrel MJ. 1997 "Risk perception and communication" in Detels
R, McEwen J, Omenn G (eds.). *Oxford Textbook of Public Health* (London: Oxford
University Press) 987-1002.

Fischhoff B, Downs J, Bruine de Bruin W. 1998 "Adolescent vulnerability: A framework for
behavioral interventions" *Applied and Preventive Psychology* 7:77-94.

Fitzgerald TE, Tennen H, Affleck G, Pransky GS. 1993 "The relative importance of dispositional optimism and control appraisals in quality of life after coronary artery bypass
surgery" *Journal of Behavioral Medicine* 16:25-43.

Ford D, Easton DF, Peto J. 1995 "Estimates of the gene frequency of $BRCA_1$ and its contribution to breast and ovarian cancer incidence" *American Journal of Human Genetics*
57:1457-1462.

Frasure-Smith N, Lesperance F, Talajic M. 1993 "Depression following myocardial infarction: Impact on 6-month survival" *Journal of the American Medical Association*
270:1819-1825.

Fredrickson BL. 1998 "What good are positive emotions?" *Review of General Psychology* 2:300-319.

Garmezy N. 1991 "Resiliency and vulnerability to adverse developmental outcomes associated with poverty" *American Behavioral Scientist* 34:416-430.

Glanz MD, Johnson JL. 1999 *Resilience and Development: Positive Life Adaptations* (New York: Kluwer Academic/Plenum).

Gottman JM, Katz LF, Hooven C. 1996 "Parental meta-emotion philosophy and and the emotional life of families: Theoretical models and preliminary data" *Journal of Family Psychology* 10:243-268.

Gould E, McEwen BS, Tanapat P, Galea LAM, Fuchs E. 1997 "Neurogenesis in the dentate gyrus of the adult tree shrew is regulated by psychosocial stress and NMDA receptor activation" *Journal of Neuroscience* 17:2492-2498.

Guralnik JM, LaCroix AZ, Abbott RD, Berkman LF, Satterfield S, Evans DA, Wallace RB. 1993 "Maintaining mobility in late life: I. Demographic characteristics and chronic conditions" *American Journal of Epidemiology* 137:845-857.

Hill JO, Peters JC. 1998 "Environmental contributions to the obesity epidemic" *Science* 280:1371-1374.

House JS, Landis KR, Umberson D. 1988 "Social relationships and health" *Science* 241:540-545.

Ickovics JR, Park CL (eds.). 1998 "Thriving: Broadening the paradigm beyond illness to health" *Journal of Social Issues* 54/2:237-244.

Institute of Medicine 1998 *Scientific Priorities and Public Values* (Washington DC: National Academy Press).

Kawachi I, Sparrow D, Spiro A, Vokonas P, Weiss ST. 1996 "A prospective study of anger and coronary heart disease: The Normative Aging Study" *Circulation* 94:2090-2095.

Kiecolt-Glaser JK, Glaser R, Gravenstein S, Malarkey WB, Sheridan J. 1996 "Chronic stress alters the immune response to influenza virus vaccine in older adults" *Proceedings of the National Academy of Sciences of the United States of America* 93:3043-3047.

Kiecolt-Glaser JK, Glaser R, Cacioppo JT, MacCallum RC, Snydersmith M, Kim C, Malarkey WB. 1997 "Marital conflict in older adults: Endocrinological and immunological correlates" *Psychosomatic Medicine* 59:339-349.

Koenig HG, George LK, Cohen HJ, Hays JC, Larson DB, Blazer DG. 1998 "The relationship between religious activities and cigarette smoking in older adults" *Journal of Gerontology* 53A:M426-M434.

Kohler CL, Davies SL, Turner-Henson A, Bailey WC. 1999 "Pulmonary disorders" in Raczynski JM, DiClemente RJ (eds.). *Handbook of Health Promotion and Disease Prevention* (New York: Kluwer Academic/Plenum Publishers) 335-348.

LaCroix AZ, Guralnik JM, Berkman LF, Wallace RB, Satterfield S. 1993 "Maintaining mobility in late life: II. Smoking, alcohol consumption, physical activity, and body mass index" *American Journal of Epidemiology* 137:858-869.

Lee CK, Klopp RG, Weindruch R, Prolla TA. 1999 "Gene expression profile of aging and its retardation by caloric restriction" *Science* 285:1390-1393.

Leedham B, Meyerowitz BE, Muirhead J, Frist WH. 1995 "Positive expectations predict health after heart transplantation" *Health Psychology* 14:74-79.

Leshner AI. 1999 "Introduction" in Glantz MD, Johnson JL (eds.). *Resilience and Development: Positive Life Adaptations* (New York: Kluwer Academic/Plenum Publishers) 1-4.

Manton KG, Corder L, Stallard E. 1997 "Chronic disability trends in the elderly U.S. populations, 1982-1994" *Proceedings of the National Academy of Sciences of the United States of America* 94:2593-2598.

McEwen BS, Stellar E. 1993 "Stress and the individual: Mechanism leading to disease" *Archives of Internal Medicine* 153:2093-2101.

Merz JF, Fischhoff B, Mazur DJ, Fischbeck PS. 1993 "A decision-analytic approach to developing standards of disclosure for medical informed consent" *Journal of Products and Toxics Liability* 15/3:191-215.

Millstein SG, Petersen AC, Nightingale EO (eds.). 1993 *Promoting the Health of Adolescents: New Directions for the Twentieth Century* (New York: Oxford University Press).

Mokdad A, Serdula MK, Dietz WH, Bowman BA, Marks JS, Koplan JP. 1999 "The spread of the obesity epidemic in the United States, 1991-1998" *Journal of the American Medical Association* 282:1519-1522.

National Advisory Mental Health Council. 1998 *Priorities for Prevention Research at NIMH* Workgroup on Mental Disorders Prevention Research, National Institute of Mental Health, National Institutes of Health (Washington DC: U.S. Department of Health and Human Services).

National Heart, Lung, and Blood Institute (NHLBI) 1998 *Behavioral Research in Cardiovascular, Lung, and Blood Health and Disease* (Washington DC: U.S. Department of Health and Human Services).

National Institute of Mental Health. 1995 *Basic Behavioral Science Research for Mental Health: A National Investment* (Washington DC: U.S. Department of Health and Human Services).

National Research Council. 1989 *Improving Risk Communication* (Washington DC: National Academy Press).

Neeper SA, Gómez-Pinilla F, Choi J, Cotman C. 1995 "Exercise and brain neurotrophins" *Nature* 373:109.

Raczynski JM, DiClemente RJ (eds.). 1999 *Handbook of Health Promotion and Disease Prevention* (New York: Kluwer Academic/Plenum Publishers).

Raczynski JM, Phillips MM, Cornell CE, Gilliland MJ, Sanderson B, Bittner V. 1999 "Cardiovascular diseases" in Raczynski JM, DiClemente RJ (eds.). *Handbook of Health Promotion and Disease Prevention* (New York: Kluwer Academic/Plenum Publishers) 231-261.

Ramey CT, Ramey SL. 1998 "Early intervention and early experience" *American Psychologist* 53:109-120.

Räukkönen K, Matthews KA, Flory JD, Owens JF, Gump BB. 1999 "Effects of optimism, pessimism, and trait anxiety on ambulatory blood pressure and mood during everyday life" *Journal of Personality and Social Psychology* 76:104-113.

Reed GM, Kemeny ME, Taylor SE, Wang H-YJ, Visscher BR. 1994 "'Realistic acceptance as a predictor of decreased survival time in gay men with AIDS" *Health Psychology* 13:299-307.

Reynolds KD, Kratt PP, Winders SE, Waterbor JW, Shuster JL Jr, Gardner MM, Harrison RA. 1999 "Cancer prevention and control" in Raczynski JM, DiClemente RJ (eds.). *Handbook of Health Promotion and Disease Prevention* (New York: Kluwer Academic/Plenum Publishers) 261-286.

Rich S (ed.). 1998 *World Symposium on Primary Pulmonary Hypertension*, Evian, France, Sept. 6-10. World Health Organization Executive Summary, pp. 1-28.

Risch N, DeLeon D, Ozelius L, Kramer P, Almasy L, Singer B, Fahn S, Breakefield X, Bressman S. 1995 "Genetic analyses of idiopathic torsion dystonia in Ashkenazi Jews and their recent descent from a small founder population" *Nature Genetics* 9:152-159.

Rose GA. 1992 *The Strategy of Preventive Medicine* (Oxford: Oxford University Press).

Rothman AJ, Kiviniemi MT. 1999 "Treating people with information: Analysis and review of approaches to communicating health risk information" *Journal of National Cancer Institute Monographs* 25:44-51.

Russek LG, Schwartz GE. 1997 "Feelings of parental caring predict health status in midlife: A 35-year follow-up of the Harvard Mastery of Stress Study" *Journal of Behavioral Medicine* 20:1-13.

Rutter M. 1990 "Psychosocial resilience and protective mechanisms" in Rolf JE, Masten AS, Cicchetti D, Neuchterlein KH, Weintraub S (eds.). *Risk and Protective Factors in the Development of Psychopathology* (New York: Cambridge University Press) 181-214.

Ryff CD, Singer B. 1998a. "The contours of positive human health" *Psychological Inquiry* 9:1-28.

Ryff CD, Singer B. 1998b. "Human health: New directions for the next millennium" *Psychological Inquiry* 9:69-85.

Ryff CD, Singer B. 2000. "Interpersonal flourishing: A positive health agenda for the new millennium" *Personality and Social Psychology Review* 4:30-44.

Ryff CD, Singer B, Love GD, Essex MJ. 1998 "Resilience in adulthood and later life: Defining features and dynamic processes" in Lomranz J (ed.). *Handbook of Aging and Mental Health: An Integrative Approach* (New York: Plenum Press) 69-96.

Sanderson BK, Taylor HA Jr. 1999 "Physical activity" in Raczynski JM, DiClemente RJ (eds.). *Handbook of Health Promotion and Disease Prevention* (New York: Kluwer Academic/Plenum Publishers) 191-206.

Scheier MF, Carver CS. 1992 "Effects of optimism on psychological and physical well-being: Theoretical overview and empirical update" *Cognitive Therapy and Research* 16:201-228.

Schumacher JE, Milby JB. 1999 "Alcohol and drug abuse" in Raczynski JM, DiClemente RJ (eds.). *Handbook of Health Promotion and Disease Prevention* (New York: Kluwer Academic/Plenum Publishers) 207-230.

Seeman TE. 1996 "Social ties and health: The benefits of social integration" *Annals of Epidemiology* 6:442-451.

Seeman TE, Singer B, Rowe JW, Horwitz RI, McEwen BS. 1997 "The price of adaptation—Allostatic load and its health consequences: MacArthur studies of successful aging" *Archives of Internal Medicine* 157:2259-2268.

Singer B, Manton KG. 1998 "The effects of health changes on projections of health service needs for the elderly population of the U.S." *Proceedings of the National Academy of Sciences of the United States of America* 95:15618-15622.

Singer B, Ryff CD. 1999. "Hierarchies of life histories and associated health risks" *Annals of the New York Academy of Sciences* 896:96-115.

Spear BA, Reinold C. 1999 "Obesity and nutrition" in Raczynski JM, DiClemente RJ (eds.). *Handbook of Health Promotion and Disease Prevention* (New York: Kluwer Academic/Plenum Publishers) 171-190.

Spiegel D. 1993 "Psychosocial intervention in cancer" *Journal of the National Cancer Institute* 85:1198-1205.

Spiegel D, Kimerling R. In press "Group psychotherapy for women with breast cancer: Relationships among social support, emotional expression, and survival" in Ryff CD, Singer B (eds.). *Emotion, Social Relationships, and Health.* (New York: Oxford University Press).

Spiegel D, Sephton SE, Terr AL, Stites DP. 1998 "Effects of psychosocial treatment in prolonging cancer survival may be mediated by neuroimmune pathways" *Annals of the New York Academy of Sciences* 840:674-683.

Staudinger UM, Marsiske M, Baltes PB. 1995 "Resilience and reserve capacity in later adulthood: Potentials and limits of development across the life span" in Cicchetti D, Cohen DJ (eds.). *Developmental Psychopathology, Vol. 2: Risk, Disorder, and Adaptation* (New York: Wiley) 801-847.

Svenson O. 1978 "Risks of road transportation from a psychological perspective" *Accident Analysis and Prevention* 10:267-280.

Taubes G. 1998 "As obesity rates rise, experts struggle to explain why" *Science* 280:1367-1368.

Taylor SE, Kemeny ME, Reed GM, Bower JE, Gruenewald TL. 2000. "Psychological resources, positive illusions, and health" *American Psychologist* 55/1:99-109.

Thoits PA. 1994 "Stressors and problem-solving: The individual as a psychological activist" *Journal of Health and Social Behavior* 35:143-159.

Todd J. 1999 "Why are certain diseases common and complicated?" *Wellcome Trust Genome Campus Symposium*, Session III, pp.1-4. Oxford, U.K.

Uchino BN, Cacioppo JT, Kiecolt-Glaser JK. 1996 "The relationship between social support and physiological processes: A review with emphasis on underlying mechanisms and implications for health" *Psychological Bulletin* 119:488-531.

Uvnäs-Moberg K. 1997 "Physiological and endocrine effects of social contact" *Annals of the New York Academy of Sciences* 807:146-163.

Uvnäs-Moberg K. 1998 "Oxytocin may mediate the benefits of positive social interaction and emotions" *Psychoneuroendocrinology* 23:819-835.

van Praag H, Kempermann G, Gage FH. 1999 "Running increases cell proliferation and neurogenesis in the adult mouse dentate gyrus" *Nature Neuroscience* 2:266-270.

Weindruch R. 1996 "Caloric restriction and aging" *Scientific American* 274:46-52.

Weinstein ND. 1998 "Accuracy of smokers' risk perceptions" *Annals of Behavioral Medicine* 20:135-140.

Werner EE, Smith RS. 1992 *Overcoming the Odds: High Risk Children from Birth to Adulthood* (Ithaca NY: Cornell University Press).

Wickelgren I. 1998 "Obesity: How big a problem?" *Science* 280:1364-1367.

Winders SE, Kohler CL, Grimley DM, Gallagher EA. 1999 "Tobacco use prevention and cessation" in Raczynski JM, DiClemente RJ (eds.). *Handbook of Health Promotion and Disease Prevention* (New York: Kluwer Academic/Plenum Publishers) 149-170.

Woloshin S, Schwartz LM. 1999 "How can we help people make sense of medical data?" *Effective Clinical Practice* 2:176-183.

Wong PTP, Fry PS. 1998 *The Human Quest for Meaning: A Handbook of Psychological Research and Clincal Applications* (Mahwah NJ: Lawrence Erlbaum Associates).

4

Environmentally Induced
Gene Expression

Mechanistic understanding of pathways to disease and preservation of good health necessitates the study of environmentally induced gene expression. A substantial body of research reveals that specific genes can be expressed at different times in an organism's life. Whether a particular gene is expressed and the degree to which it is expressed depend strongly on the environmental conditions experienced by the organism. Such gene expression is implicated in both positive and negative health effects.

Vulnerability and resistance to disease are strongly influenced by genetic endowment and environmental conditions during early periods in development (Coplan et al., 1996; Lui et al., 1997; de Kloet et al., 1998; Laban et al., 1995; Ladd et al., 1996; Levine et al., 1967; Meaney et al., 1991; Plotsky and Meaney, 1993; Seckl and Meaney, 1993). At each stage, development is promoted by the activation of specific genes that regulate cellular activity, migration, and differentiation. This occurs, however, within environmental contexts that shape the processes underlying various stages of an organism's development. At its most fundamental level, development is a constant interaction between environmental and genetic factors.

Genes exert their influence by encoding proteins. The level of such gene activity, however, is a regulated process. As molecules, genes are subject to regulation by intracellular factors that, in turn, are a reflection of environmental factors. Neither genes nor environment dominates development; rather there is continual interaction between genes and the environment. Phenotype emerges as a function of this constant dialogue, and any effort to ascribe percentage values to isolated variables is likely to be biologically meaningless.

The critical questions in this arena concern gene expression. Studies of gene expression focus on the regulation of gene activity and the mechanisms of gene-environment interactions. The human genome project and the recent development of microarray chip technologies offer researchers remarkable tools for examining the development of vulnerability or resistance to disease. Microarray chips are thin wafers, approximately the size of a dime, containing a densely packed, orderly arrangement of thousands of different probes, utilized for matching known and unknown DNA samples. The technology monitors an entire genome on a single chip, thereby facilitating the detection of gene expression with unprecedented resolution (Ekins and Chu, 1999; Schena, 2000). Realizing the full potential of whole genome analyses will require multidisciplinary research projects that integrate molecular biology with physiology and the behavioral and social sciences. As modern genetics identifies individual or multiple genes associated with many human diseases, such advances will only underscore the importance of understanding the environmental factors that regulate expression of these and other genes.

Scientifically, the key task is to define the pathways that lead to disease. This requires understanding first how genes and related factors might be associated with the onset of particular disease outcomes and, second, tracking relevant mediating conditions. The behavioral and social sciences are essential to advancing knowledge of these environmental conditions. Full explication of health pathways thus hinges on integrative multidisciplinary research.

In the subsections that follow we present examples illustrative of the current evidential base that connects behavior and the social environment to gene expression (direct and indirect) and subsequent pathways to health outcomes. As a collectivity, these examples represent a coarse-grained description of what is, in fact, a dynamic process of interrelationships between social and physical environments and complex patterns of gene expression that operate over the entire lifetime of different organisms. The examples are each suggestive of new research directions that, if pursued, would notably enhance understanding of pathways to health outcomes.

GENE EXPRESSION AND PRENATAL DEVELOPMENT

Prenatal life represents a period of cell division and differentiation, the result of which is tissue formation and function. Development is costly in metabolic terms, requiring massive amounts of energy reserves to fuel the growth of bone, muscle, brain cells, and so on. The mother is the sole source of nutrients for this development, and the interplay between the mother and the fetus is reflected in placental function. Demanding conditions experienced by the mother are transmitted to the fetus through endocrine and nutritional signals. These signals result in both short-term and long-term changes in gene expression in the fetus (Roberts and Redman, 1993; Wadhwa, 1998). Thus, the origins of adult disease are often found in prenatal life.

An example of this phenomenon, where behavioral characteristics of the mother are also relevant is interuterine growth retardation (IUGR; Sattar et al., 1999; de Onis et al., 1998, Gülmezouglu et al., 1997). It is estimated that genetic mutations account for approximately 10 percent of the cases of IUGR. The remainder of the cases are due to a wide range of environmental conditions, including maternal smoking, serious infection, malnutrition (especially protein deficiency), excessive alcohol consumption, abuse of drugs, and extreme maternal stress (Kramer, 1987a, b). Each of these risk factors is associated with increased risk of high levels of glucocorticoids in the mother. Glucocorticoids inhibit insulin-like growth factor (IGF) gene expression, as well as the action of IGF (de Kloet et al., 1998). They also increase the production of IGF-binding protein 1 (IGF-1), which serves to biologically inactivate IGF. Both conditions impair development and contribute to the emergence of IUGR. The alterations in gene expression accompanying IUGR increase the sensitivity of hypothalamic-pituitary-adrenal (HPA) and sympathetic responses to stress in later life (Ladd et al., 1996). The elevated levels of stress hormones, in turn, increase vulnerability of the individual to diabetes and heart disease. An important challenge for future research is to understand how psychosocial adversity over the life course of low-birth-weight babies—having experienced IUGR—is related to subsequent processes of gene expression that culminate in diabetes, coronary heart disease, or both.

PERSONAL TIES AND GENE EXPRESSION IN MIDLIFE

Increasing evidence documents the role of personal ties on gene expression in midlife. For example, the genetic transcription responsible for the production of lymphocyte growth hormone (L-GH) is, in part, age related, as L-GH secretion decreases with increasing age (Nordin and Proust, 1987; Krishnaraj et al., 1998). However, extended disruption of personal ties also modulates L-GH levels. Caregivers of spouses with Alzheimer's disease have markedly suppressed L-GH concentrations compared to age- and gender-matched controls (Wu et al., 1999). The transduction process by which disruption of personal ties modulates growth hormone (GH) messenger RNA (mRNA) is most likely to involve stress hormones such as adrenocoricotropic hormone (ACTH), cortisol, and catecholamines (Kiecolt-Glaser et al., 1997). Reduced levels of GH consequential to a disruption of personal ties can be involved in immune system function. In particular, current evidence suggests that GH promotes the efficacy of lymphocytes in responding to antigens, with its route of action being via the TH-1 and TH-2 helper cytokine system (Wu et al., 1999). Research is needed to clarify the details of this proposed process, including whether these perturbations in immune system parameters translate to downstream health outcomes. In addition, we need to understand how cumulative adversity in a variety of interpersonal relationships is connected to processes of gene expression that may culminate in impaired immune function and thereby contribute to a range of disease outcomes.

ANIMAL MODELS AND THE CONSEQUENCES OF MOTHER-CHILD INTERACTIONS

Although the above examples focus on human populations and important research agendas that follow from them, animal models have been and will continue to be a main route to achieving deeper understanding of mechanisms of gene expression. For example, the role and character of mother-child interactions that influence neural development have recently been studied in detail in rats (Lui et al., 1997; Caldji et al., 1998; Francis et al., 1999). Specifically, there are two forms of maternal behavior in the rat—licking and grooming of pups (LG) and arched-back nursing (ABN)—that appear to regulate the development of stress reactivity in the offspring. As adults the offspring of mothers exhibiting high levels of LG-ABN care showed reduced plasma ACTH and corticosterone responses to restraint stress. These animals also show significantly increased hippocampal glucocorticoid receptor mRNA expression, enhanced glucocorticoid negative feedback sensitivity, and decreased hypothalamic corticotropin-releasing hormone mRNA levels. The results of these studies suggest that the behavior of the mother toward her offspring can program the expression of genes regulating neuroendocrine response to stress in adulthood (Lui et al., 1997).

Support for this claim derives from the fact that as adults the offspring of low LG-ABN mothers exhibit increased fearfulness relative to offspring of high LG-ABN mothers (Caldji et al., 1998). They also show increased corticotropin-releasing factor (CRF) receptor levels in the locus coeruleus and decreased central benzodiazepine receptor levels in the basolateral and central nucleus of the amygdala, as well as increased CRF mRNA expression in the central amygdala. Predictably, stress-induced increases in levels of norepinephrine in the paraventricular nucleus of the hypothalamus were significantly higher in the offspring of low LG-ABN mothers (Francis et al., 1999). These are all neurophysiological signs of elevated reactivity to stress in adulthood.

It may seem surprising that rather subtle variations in maternal behavior have such profound impact on development. However, for a rat pup, the first six weeks of life do not hold a great deal of stimulus diversity. Stability is the theme of the burrow, and the social environment in the first days of life is defined by the mother and the littermates. The mother then serves as the primary link between the environment and the developing animal. Following on these results, an important line of research, linked to pathway studies in humans that are the core of this report, is identification of the features of rat life histories and their relationship to gene expression that contribute to downstream health outcomes.

INTERGENERATIONAL TRANSMISSION OF BEHAVIOR

Another line of recent animal research having profound implications for future investigations in humans centers around evidence that individual differences in maternal behavior are transmitted across generations (in both rats and nonhuman primates). For example, in rats the female offspring of high LG-ABN mothers show significantly more licking and grooming and arched-back nursing than female offspring of low LG-ABN mothers (Francis et al., 1999). In rhesus monkeys there is clear evidence for inter-generational transfer of rejection of infants by mothers. The rate of rejection of infants by mothers correlated with the rejection rates of their mothers (Suomi, 1987; Suomi and Levine, 1998). In vervet monkeys, daughters reared by mothers who consistently spent a large amount of time in physical contact with their offspring became mothers who were similarly more attentive to their offspring (Fairbanks, 1989).

An important complement to these findings is evidence indicating that specific environmental events can alter trajectories of development not only in the affected offspring but also into the next generation (Francis et al., 1999). For example, biological offspring of low LG-ABN mothers cross-fostered onto high-LG-ABN mothers are indistinguishable from the natural progeny of high-LG-ABN mothers in terms of behavioral measures of fearfulness or of HPA axis response to stressful experiences. In addition, these behavioral effects are reflected in corresponding changes in CRF gene expression in the hypothalamus and amygdala. Moreover, in adult females of both the cross-fostered and natural progeny groups, their maternal behavior was typical of high-LG-ABN mothers. Similarly, the behavior of adult offspring of high-LG-ABN mothers reared by low-LG-ABN dams resembled that of the normal offspring of low-LG-ABN mothers.

An example relating directly to predisease pathways concerns cross-fostering between borderline hypertensive rats (BHR) and wild-type WKY mothers (Gouldsborough and Ashton, 1998; Sanders and Gray, 1997; Myers et al., 1989). The starting point for this investigation is the introduction of the spontaneously hypertensive rat (SHR), a strain bred for the appearance of hypertension in adolescence. While the selective breeding implies a genetic background, the expression of the hypertensive trait is also influenced by epigenetic factors. SHR pups reared by wild-type WKY mothers do exhibit hypertension to the extent of kin reared by SHR dams. However, BHR—a hybrid formed by SHR-WKY matings—pups reared by WKY mothers do not express the spontaneous hypertensive phenotype. An important future research priority is to determine whether these effects are associated with changes in the expression of genes that regulate blood pressure. Extending the discussion to humans, it should be asked which supportive environments for which groups of people induce gene expression that reduces the risk of hypertension.

PLASTICITY OF GENETIC TRAJECTORIES

The above cross-fostering examples also serve to illustrate the adaptive value of plasticity. If a genetically determined trajectory is not advantageous, then the ability to adjust in response to a new environmental signal would have an adaptive value. These effects are not so readily seen in the wild, since low-LG-ABN rats are typically reared by low-LG-ABN mothers. Similarly in mice, BALBc pups—a strain that is normally very fearful with elevated HPA response to stress—are reared by BALBc mothers. Because parents provide both genes and environment to their biological offspring, these factors enhance the disadvantageous consequences seen in adulthood. For this reason, knowing that a mouse has a BALBc pedigree is usually sufficient to predict a high level of timidity in adulthood. BALBc mice cross-fostered to C57 mothers are significantly less fearful and have lower HPA responses to stress (Zaharia et al., 1996; Anisman et al., 1998). These examples emphasize the potential for traits to be modified by environmental interventions. They clarify that gene expression accompanies such interventions; and they emphasize the importance of pursuing analogous studies in humans with a far more diverse set of environmental influences.

Having emphasized the impact of parental care, it is important to observe that caring takes place in a great diversity of natural environments and that this added variation is consequential for development and health. Important examples of the joint influence of mother-infant bonding and other environmental factors are studies of Bonnet macaque mother-infant dyads maintained under one of three foraging conditions: low foraging demand (LFD), where food was readily available high foraging demand (HFD), where ample food was available but required long periods of searching; and variable foraging demand (VFD), a mixture of the previous two conditions on an unpredictable schedule (Andrews and Rosenblum, 1994). Prior to the time these conditions were imposed, there were no differences in the nature of mother-infant interactions. Following a number of months of the experimental conditions, however, there were highly significant differences in mother-infant interactions. The VFD condition was clearly the most disruptive. Mother-infant conflict increased under the VFD condition. Infants of mothers housed under these conditions were significantly more timid and fearful. The infants showed signs of depression commonly observed in maternally separated macaque infants, even while the infants were in contact with their mothers. As adolescents, infants reared in the VFD conditions were more fearful and submissive and showed less social play behavior.

More recent studies (Coplan et al., 1996, 1998; Rosenblum et al., 1994) show that, as adults, monkeys reared under VFD conditions have increased levels of CRF. Increased central CRF drive suggests altered noradrenergic and serotonergic responses to stress, exactly as seen in adolescent VFD-reared animals. An important research objective is to ascertain whether these traits are transmitted to the next generation. Researching predisease pathways, it is also important to document the later-life health profiles of VFD-reared and -maintained macaques in comparison with macaques reared in either of the stable environments, LFD or HFD.

WHOLE-GENOME ANALYSES

All of the studies described above provide a coarse picture of the interrelationships between environmental fluctuations, behavior, physiological response, and gene expression over the life course. To date, a limiting factor has been the absence of a technology for carrying out whole-genome studies coupled with the unavailability of whole-genome data. This situation is changing rapidly. Whole-genome data are currently available for a diversity of organisms (e.g., yeast, M. *tuberculosis*, H. *influenza*, *drosophila*, C. *elegans*), including humans.[1] The nematode C. *elegans* and *drosophila* are among the more prominent nonhuman organisms where behavioral studies have also been carried out. In addition, the development of microarray chip technology (Fodor, 1997; Cho et al., 1998; Ekins and Chu, 1999; Schena, 2000) has made studies of gene expression feasible with unprecedented precision. Over the next decade it should be possible to study environmentally induced gene expression as a dynamic process from conception to death. The greatest progress and short-term payoff are likely to be in animal studies (Lee et al., 1999); however, studies in humans are already clarifying pathways to cancers (Golub et al., 1999; Alon et al., 1999) and pulmonary fibrosis (Kaminski et al., 2000) with unprecedented

---

[1] The data are available electronically at www.nhgri.nih.gov/PMGifs/Genomes/allorg.html.

precision. This implies that many of the questions documented in this report regarding predisease pathways, positive health, inequalities, and community-level influences should be answerable in animal populations down to the level of gene expression. Such studies should stimulate a host of investigations on human populations that will provide a deeply more integrated understanding of pathways to diverse health outcomes.

RECOMMENDATIONS

NIH should support integrative research aimed at understanding the role of environmentally induced gene expression in disease etiology and promotion of health. This initiative should include:

- studies that combine environmental manipulations with physiological and molecular assessments to provide refined understanding of conditions leading to dysfunction and the mechanisms that preserve allostasis;
- studies that explore in animal models the relationships between chronic stress, interactions among intervening systems (e.g., HPA axis and immune systems), and health outcomes;
- initiation of studies using microarray chip technologies to monitor gene expression associated with a broad range of environmental manipulations;
- development of animal housing facilities, particularly for rodents, that more closely approximate species-specific natural habitats.

REFERENCES

Alon U, Barkai N, Notterman DA, Gish K, Ybarra S, Mack D, Levine AJ. 1999 "Patterns of gene expression revealed by clustering analysis of tumor and normal colon tissues probed by oligonucleotide arrays" *Proceedings of the National Academy of Sciences of the United States of America* 96:6745-6750.

Andrews MW, Rosenblum LA. 1994 "The development of affiliative and agonistic social patterns in differentially reared monkeys" *Child Development* 65/5:1398-1404.

Anisman H, Zaharia MD, Meaney MJ, Merali Z. 1998 "Do early-life events permanently alter behavioral and hormonal responses to stressors?" *International Journal of Developmental Neuroscience* 16/3-4:149-164.

Caldji C, Tannenbaum B, Sharma S, Francis D, Plotsky PM, Meaney MJ. 1998 "Maternal care during infancy regulates the development of neural systems mediating the expression of fearfulness in the rat" *Proceedings of the National Academy of Sciences of the United States of America* 95:5335-5340.

Cho RJ, Fromont-Racene M, Wodicka L, Feierbach B, Stearns T, Legrain P, Lockhart DJ, Davis R. 1998 "Parallel analysis of genetic selections using whole genome oligonucleotide arrays" *Proceedings of the National Academy of Sciences of the United States of America* 95:3752-3757.

Coplan JD, Andrews MW, Rosenblum LA, Owens MJ, Friedman S, Gorman JM, Nemeroff CB. 1996 "Persistent elevations of cerebrospinal fluid concentrations of corticotropin-releasing factor in adult nonhuman primates exposed to early-life stressors: Implications for the pathophysiology of mood and anxiety disorders" *Proceedings of the National Academy of Sciences of the United States of America* 93/4:1619-1623.

Coplan JE, Trost RC, Owens MJ, Cooper TB, Gorman JM, Nemeroff CB, Rosenblum LA. 1998 "Cerebrospinal fluid concentrations of somatostatin and biogenic amines in grown primates reared by mothers exposed to manipulated foraging conditions" *Archives of General Psychiatry* 55:473-477.

de Kloet ER, Vreugdenhil E, Oitzl MS, Joëls M. 1998 "Brain corticosteriod receptor balance in health and disease" *Endocrine Reviews* 19/3:269-301.

de Onis M, Villar J, Gülmezouglu M. 1998 "Nutritional interventions to prevent interuterine growth retardation: Evidence from randomized controlled trials" *European Journal of Clinical Nutrition* 52:S83-S93.

Ekins R, Chu FW. 1999 "Microarrays: Their origins and application" *Trends in Biotechnology* 17:217-218.

Fairbanks LA. 1989 "Early experience and cross-generational continuity of mother-infant contact in vervet monkeys" *Developmental Psychobiology* 22/7:669-681.

Fodor SA. 1997 "Massively parallel genomics" *Science* 277:393-395.

Francis D, Diorio J, Liu D, Meaney MJ. 1999 "Nongenetic transmission across generations of maternal behavior and stress responses in the rat" *Science* 286:1155-1158.

Golub TR, Slonim DK, Tamaya P, Huard C, Gaasenbeek M, Mesirov JP, Coller H, Loh L, Downing JR, Caliguiri MA, Bloomfield CD, Lander ES. 1999 "Molecular classification of cancer: Class discovery and class prediction by gene expression monitoring" *Science* 286:531-537.

Gouldsborough I, Ashton N. 1998 "Effect of cross-fostering on neonatal sodium balance and adult blood pressure in the spontaneously hypertensive rat" *Clinical Experiments in Pharmacological Physiology* 25/12:1024-1031.

Gülmezouglu M, de Onis M, Villar J. 1997 "Effectiveness of interventions to prevent or treat impaired fetal growth" *Obstetric Gynecology Survey* 52:139-149.

Kaminski N, Allard JD, Pittet JF, Zuo F, Griffiths MJD, Morris D, Huang X, Sheppard D, Heller RA. 2000 "Global analysis of gene expression in pulmonary fibrosis reveals distinct programs regulating lung inflammation and fibrosis" *Proceedings of the National Academy of Sciences of the United States of America* 97:1778-1783.

Kiecolt-Glaser JK, Glaser R, Cacioppo JT, MacCallum RC, Snydersmith M, Kim C, Malarkey WB. 1997 "Marital conflict in older adults: Endocrinological and immunological correlates" *Psychosomatic Medicine* 59/4:339-349.

Kramer MS. 1987a "Determinants of low birthweight: Methodological assessment and meta analysis" *Bulletin of the World Health Organization* 65/5:663-737.

Kramer MS. 1987b "Interuterine growth retardation and gestational duration determinants" *Pediatrics* 80/4:502-511.

Krishnaraj R, Zaks A, Unterman T. 1998 "Relationship between plasma IGF-I levels, in vitro correlates of immunity, and human senescence" *Clinical Immunology and Immunopathology* 88/3:264-270.

Laban O, Markovic BM, Dimitrijevic M, Jankovic BD. 1995 "Maternal deprivation and early weaning modulate experimental allergic encephalomyelitis in the rat" *Brain, Behavior, and Immunity* 9:9-19.

Ladd CO, Owens MJ, Nemeroff CB. 1996 "Persistent changes in corticotropin-releasing factor neuronal systems induced by maternal deprivation" *Endocrinology* 137/4:1212-1218.

Lee C-K, Klopp RG, Weindruch R, Prollo TA. 1999 "Gene expression profile of aging and its retardation by caloric restriction" *Science* 285:1390-1393.

Levine S, Haltmeyer GC, Karas G, Denenberg VH. 1967 "Physiological and behavioral effects of infantile stimulation" *Physiology and Behavior* 2:55-59.

Lui D, Diorio J, Tannenbaum B, Caldji C, Francis D, Freedman A, Sharma S, Pearson D, Plotsky PM, Meaney MJ. 1997 "Maternal care, hippocampal glucocorticoid receptors, and hypothalamic-pituitary-adrenal response to stress" *Science* 277:1659-1662.

Meaney MJ, Aitken DH, Bhatnagar S, Sapolsky RM. 1991 "Postnatal handling attenuates certain neuroendocrine, anatomical, and cognitive dysfunctions associated with aging in female rats" *Neurobiology of Aging* 12:31-38.

Myers MM, Brunelli SA, Shair HN, Squire JM, Hofer MA. 1989 "Relationships between maternal behavior of SHR and WKY dams and adult blood pressures of cross-fostered F1 pups" *Developmental Psychobiology* 22/1:55-67.

Nordin AA, Proust JJ. 1987 "Signal transduction mechanisms in the immune system: Potential implication in immunosenescence" *Endocrinology and Metabolism Clinics of North America* 16/4:919-945.

Plotsky PM, Meaney MJ. 1993 "Early, postnatal experience alters hypothalamic corticotropin-releasing factor (CRF) mRNA, median eminence CRF content and stress-induced release in adult rats" *Molecular Brain Research* 18:195-200.

Roberts JM, Redman CWG. 1993 "Pre-eclampsia: More than pregnancy-induced hypertension" *Lancet* 341:1447-1451.

Rosenblum L, Coplan J, Friedman S, Bassoff T, Gorman J, Andrews M. 1994 "Adverse early experiences affect noradrenergic and serotonergic functioning in adult primates" *Biological Psychiatry* 35:221-227.

Sanders BJ, Gray MJ. 1997 "Early environmental influences can attenuate the blood pressure response to acute stress in borderline hypertensive rats" *Physiological Behavior* 61/5:749-754.

Sattar N, Greer IA, Galloway PJ, Packard CJ, Shepherd J, Kelly, T, Mathers A. 1999 "Lipid and lipoprotein concentrations in pregnancies complicated by intrauterine growth restriction *Journal of Clinical Endocrinology and Metabolism* 84:128-130.

Schena M (ed.). 2000 *Microarray Biochip Technology* (Natick MA: Eaton Publishing).

Seckl JR, Meaney MJ. 1993 "Early life events and later development of ischaemic heart disease" *The Lancet* 342/13:1236.

Suomi SJ. 1987 "Genetic and maternal contributions to individual differences in rhesus monkey biobehavioral development" in Krasnegor NA, Blass EM, Hofer MA, Smotherman WP (eds.). *Perinatal Development: A Psychobiological Perspective* (New York: Academic Press) 397-420.

Suomi SJ, Levine S. 1998 "Psychobiology of intergenerational effects of trauma: Evidence from animal studies" in Danieli Y (ed.). *Intergenerational Handbook of Multigenerational Legacies* (New York: Plenum Press) 623-637.

Wadhwa PD. 1998 "Pre-natal stress and life-time development" in Friedman HS (ed.). *Encyclopedia of Mental Health* (San Diego CA: Academic Press).

Wu H, Wang J, Cacioppo JT, Glaser R, Kiecolt-Glaser JK, Malarkey WB. 1999 "Chronic stress associated with spousal caregiving of patients with Alzheimer's dementia is associated with downregulation of B-lymphocyte GH mRNA" *Journal of Gerontology, Series A, Biological Sciences and Medical Sciences* 54/4:M212-M215.

Zaharia MD, Shanks N, Meaney MJ, Anisman H. 1996 "The effects of early postnatal stimulation on Morris water-maze acquisition in adult mice: Genetic and maternal factors" *Psychopharmacology* 128:227-239.

5

Personal Ties

The preceding discussions of predisease pathways, positive health, and environmentally induced gene expression emphasize the importance of proximate social interactions. Understanding the mediating and moderating effects of personal ties on mental and physical functioning is necessary to elucidate fully the mechanisms underlying health and disease. Social factors, for instance, are capable of activating aspects of innate or natural immunity that are the earliest responses to infectious or inflammatory responses (Maier and Watkins, 1998), and social influences on gene expression have been demonstrated (Gottlieb, 1998; Wu et al., 1999).

THE CENTRALITY OF PERSONAL TIES

Personal ties are a ubiquitous part of life, serving important social, psychological, and behavioral functions across the life span (see Cacioppo et al., in press a). People form personal ties with others from the moment they are born. The survival of newborns depends on their attachment to and nurturance by others over an extended period of time (Baumeister and Leary, 1995). The human brain has evolved to recognize faces holistically (Farah et al., 1998). Distress vocalization, a signaling mechanism designed to solicit and sustain parental caring, is one of the most primitive forms of audiovocal communication. Language, the bedrock of complex social interaction, is universal in humans. Even in the rare instances in which human language is not modeled or taught, a language system develops nevertheless (Goldin-Meadow and Mylander, 1983). Evolution, it appears, has sculpted the human genome to be sensitive to and succoring of contact and relationships with others.

The need to belong does not stop at infancy; rather affiliation and nurturant social relationships are essential for physical and psychological well-being across the life span (Gardner et al., 2000; Seeman, 1996; Cohen and Syme, 1985). Affirmative social interactions—those satisfying needs for autonomy, competence, and relatedness—are related to feeling understood and appreciated (Reis, in press), and emotional disclosure improves affect and physical functioning among rheumatoid arthritis patients (Kelley et al., 1997). Disruptions of personal ties, whether through ridicule, discrimination, separation, divorce, or bereavement, are among the most stressful events people must endure (Gardner et al., 2000). Models of mental illness suggest that biological events (e.g., genetic heritage, in utero insult) produce a susceptibility to severe mental illness, but it is this vulnerability combined with the stress of life events, especially social events, that produces mood disorders, psychotic symptoms, or social apathy in late adolescence or early adulthood. Cognitive and interpersonal deficits in childhood and adolescence can further impair individuals from learning social and instrumental skills that help them avoid life stressors and achieve age-appropriate social roles. In sum, inadequate and restricted social connection during infancy and childhood has dramatic effects on psychopathology across the life span.

Relationships in adult life have been studied for their contributions to intimacy (Berscheid and Reis, 1998) and well-being (Myers and Diener, 1995; Ryff and Singer, 2000; Sternberg and Hojaat, 1997) as well as the adverse consequences of divorce and bereavement (Kiecolt-Glaser et al., 1998), deficits in belongingness (Baumeister and Leary, 1995), and dispositional and cognitive factors contributing to loneliness and depression (Cacioppo et al., in press b; Marangoni and Ickes, 1989). Studies show that marital dysfunction and conflict have significant physiological consequences. A study of older adults and long-term marriages showed that 30 minutes of conflict discussion was associated with increases in cortisol, adrenocorticotropic hormone, and norepinephrine in women but not in men (Kiecolt-Glaser et al., 1997). Other studies have linked marital conflict with high blood pressure (Ewart et al., 1991), elevated plasma catecholamine levels (Malarkey et al., 1994), and autonomic activation (Levenson et al., 1993).

Family life can also contribute to stress and dysfunctional coping with consequences for detrimental health behaviors (e.g., smoking, sedentary lifestyles, poor eating habits, type A behavior patterns). Characteristics of the family environment that may undermine the health of children and adolescents include a social climate that is conflictual and angry or even violent and abusive; parent-child relationships that are unresponsive and lacking in cohesiveness, warmth, and emotional support; and parenting styles that are either overly controlling and dominating or involved with little imposition of rules and structure (Taylor et al., 1997). Empirical evidence suggests that long-term exposure to such conditions contributes to deficits in emotional understanding, difficulties with appropriate expression of emotion, increased emotional reactivity to conflict, and maladaptive coping strategies for managing stressful events more generally (Repetti et al., in press).

Apart from family life, the social world also involves comparisons and standards that may be consequential for health. In the traditional culture of Fiji, the ideal body is robust, but satellite TV brought shows to Fijians that featured svelte women. In a 1995-1998 survey, teen Fijian girls who watched TV at least three nights per week were 50 percent more likely than others to report feeling too big or fat and were 30 percent more likely to diet even though the more frequent TV watchers were not more overweight. Fifteen percent said they had vomited to control their weight, up from 3 percent in 1995, and the proportion who scored high on risk for disordered eating was 29 percent in 1998, in contrast to 13 percent in 1995 (Becker, 1999).

At the population level of analysis, epidemiological studies have shown that social isolation is a major risk factor for morbidity and mortality from widely varying causes (Berkman and Syme, 1979; Berkman and Breslow, 1983; House et al., 1988; Seeman et al., 1993). This relationship is evident even after statistically controlling for known biological risk factors, social status, and baseline measures of health. Astonishingly, the strength of social isolation as a risk factor is comparable to high blood pressure, obesity, sedentary lifestyles, and possibly even smoking (House et al., 1988). Increased survival has been associated with high quantity or quality of social relationships in several prospective studies (Funch and Marshall, 1983; Joffres et al., 1985; Rodin, 1986; Goodwin et al., 1987; Ganster and Victor, 1988; Kennedy et al., 1988; House et al., 1994). Women not socially isolated were at substantially lower risk for dying of cancer (Reynolds and Kaplan, 1990), and married cancer patients survived longer than unmarried persons (Goodwin et al., 1987). Emotional support is associated with longer survival following breast, colorectal, or lung cancer (Ell et al., 1992).

Being part of a social network, however, can have detrimental as well as salubrious effects. Membership in networks, for example, provides access to domestic, economic, and informational resources (Uehara, 1990). The value to the individual of such ties, however, depends on the character of the network. If one's ties are limited to a tightly knit group, the resources available through that group, especially informational resources, are likely to be limited, whereas ties to others who are otherwise unconnected expands the potential resource base (Pescosolido, 1986, 1991; Uehara, 1990).

A final realm of relevant research pertains to the experimental literature in animals, where possible confounds can be better controlled. Here the absence or impairment of personal ties has been associated with altered physiological responses. In a series of studies in cynomolgus monkeys, experimentally induced social disruptions and instability were found to promote coronary atherogenesis (Manuck et al., 1995; Skantze et al., 1998). Animals exhibiting a heightened cardiac reactivity to stress developed the most extensive coronary lesions. Disruptions of personal ties were further shown to increase the formation of endothelial lesions even in the absence of an atherosclerosis-inducing diet (Skantze et al., 1998). On the positive side, animal studies also clarify the neurobiology of affiliation and attachment (Panksepp, 1998). A review of caregiver-infant and adult-adult (heterosexual) pair bonds showed recurrent associations between high levels of activity in the hypothalamic-pituitary-adrenal (HPA) axis and subsequent expression of social behaviors and attachments (Carter, 1998). Central neuropeptides, especially oxytocin and vasopressin, are implicated in social bonding and central control of the HPA axis. Moreover, in both male and female rats, oxytocin exerts potent antistress effects, such as decreases in blood pressure, heart rate, and cortisol levels, with effects lasting from one to several weeks (Uvnäs-Moberg, 1997, 1998; Petersson et al., 1996).

Together, these human and animal studies provide extensive evidence of linkages between the social relational realm and health. Some focus on proximal social ties and their implications for health behaviors, while others examine the neurobiology of interpersonal conflict or relational intimacy. Still other inquiries document, via large epidemiological samples, links between social integration or isolation and unfolding profiles of morbidity and mortality. How the social world is structured by community environments (see Chapter 6) and macro-level influences (see Chapter 8) is also a key target for future inquiries. A major message is that all such levels of analysis are necessary to fully explicate how personal ties impact health. The mechanisms underlying these effects cannot be fully explicated by biological, behavioral, or social approaches alone but rather require multilevel integrative analyses.

The following sections describe areas of particular importance in advancing this broad agenda. Key future directions pertain to studies of how personal ties influence genetic expression as well as brain structure and function and neuroimmunological activity. The links between social factors and infectious disease are also considered. A final section underscores the need to connect the extensive epidemiological literature on social support and health to the mechanisms (behavioral, neurobiological) through which these effects occur.

PERSONAL TIES AND GENE EXPRESSION

As described in Chapter 4, extended disruption of personal ties, such as that experienced by people caring for their spouses with Alzheimer's disease, results in significant suppression of lymphocyte growth hormone (L-GH; Wu et al., 1999). It is likely that this suppression is due to the effects of stress hormones and catecholamines on gene expression (Malarkey et al., 1996) and may compromise immune function.

The social influence on gene expressions is also illustrated in recent research on early nurturance. Rhesus monkeys characterized by high hypothalamic-pituitary-adrenal (HPA) reactivity have a lower threshold for stress reactions and show larger responses to stressors than their genetically less reactive counterparts. The mothers of low- and high-reactive monkeys also differ in their attention to and nurturance of their infants, with the mothers of high-reactive monkeys being less attentive and nurturant. Cross-fostering, however, influences the phenotypic expression of these genotypes: High-reactive infants raised by low-reactive mothers produce adults who are low in stress reactivity. Thus, HPA reactivity is a genetically inherited trait, but high reactivity can be controlled by modifying personal ties during development (Suomi, 1999; see Chapter 2).

Research further shows that early tactile deprivation reduces the number of glucocorticoid receptor binding sites in the hippocampus and frontal cortex via an action on gene expression (Meaney et al., 1985). Studies of rat pups show that transient early life stress (e.g., brief handling) attenuates the behavioral and neuroendocrine responses to stressors encountered in adulthood, whereas more severe early life stressors (e.g., protracted separation from the dam) accentuate responses to these stressors in adulthood (Anisman et al., 1998). These early life experiences particularly affect HPA functioning, which can modify the responses to subsequent stressors. These effects again appear to be mediated by variations in maternal care. Cross-fostering with mothers who exhibited more licking and grooming and nurturance of pups during the first 10 days of life revealed reduced adrenocorticotropic hormone and corticosterone responses to acute stress. As mothers these rats also tended to lick and groom their pups (Liu et al., 1997; see Chapter 4). Collectively, these studies illustrate the reciprocal influences between the social and biological factors in health and, in so doing, reframe the guiding questions as fundamentally about the roles of nature and nurture.

PERSONAL TIES AND BRAIN FUNCTION AND STRUCTURE

Personal ties constitute a major influence on the emotions of an individual, which are increasingly recognized to be important for fundamental tasks of survival and adaptation (Damasio, 1994; Pinker, 1997; Ekman and Davidson, 1994). In addition, plasticity in the neural circuitry underlying emotion plays an important role in the influence of early environmental factors on later behaviors and psychopathological susceptibility (Meaney et al., 1996).

Research demonstrates a number of ways that emotions affect brain functioning. For example, positive affective states induced by viewing film clips increases left-side prefrontal and anterior temporal activation, whereas induced negative affect elicits an opposite pattern of asymmetric activation (Davidson et al., 1990). The right inferior region and the right medial orbital region of the prefrontal cortex have been found to be activated more strongly among individuals exhibiting anxiety disorders than among controls not exhibiting psychopathology (Rauch et al., 1997). Studies of patients with selective bilateral destruction in the amygdala suggest the importance of this brain region for specific tasks involving emotional processing (Davidson et al., 2000).

From a developmental perspective, brain electrical measures of baseline prefrontal activation asymmetry show little stability between the ages of 3 and 11 (Davidson and Rickman, 1999), a period during which the central circuitry of emotion, particularly in the prefrontal cortex, is still undergoing development (Huttenlocher, 1990). Emotions also can affect the development of specific brain regions. As already discussed, the early interactions between rat pups and their mothers—frequency of maternal licking/grooming and arched-backed nursing—and the resulting biological changes affect the pups' response to stress stimuli as adults. In addition, these offspring show increased central benzodiazepine receptor densities in parts of the amygdala and in the locus coeruleus (LC), increased density of corticosteriod receptors in the LC, and decreased corticotropin-releasing hormone receptor density in the LC (Caldji et al., 1998). They also show increased concentrations of receptors for glucocorticoids in both the hippocampus and the prefrontal cortex (Liu et al., 1997; Meaney et al., 1996).

Rhesus monkeys exposed to a human intruder who appears in profile (i.e., makes no eye contact) freeze more frequently and for longer duration than do animals at which the intruder stares (Kalin et al., 1998). A few animals, however, display levels of freezing during the stare condition that are indistinguishable from their freezing during the no-eye-contact condition. These animals show more extreme patterns of prefrontal cortex activation asymmetry and cortisol levels than their counterparts. Behavioral differences that help account for some of the variance in base levels of prefrontal activation asymmetry and cortisol levels were revealed only when behavior under exceptional conditions was assessed (Kalin et al., 2000). Individuals who habitually fail to regulate their affective responses in a context-sensitive situation may have functional impairment of the hippocampus and/or stria terminalis (Davidson et al., 2000).

Collectively, such findings highlight the plasticity of certain regions of the brain and raise the possibility that social and behavioral interventions, even those occurring during adulthood, can not only affect neural function but also influence neurogenesis. Critical for future research are inquiries working at the nexus of social interaction, emotion, and brain activity. The growing field of affective neuroscience (Davidson, 1998; Panksepp, 1998) is well poised to make major contributions to such integrative initiatives.

PERSONAL TIES AND NEUROIMMUNOLOGICAL ACTIVITY

Empirical observations of social influences on autonomic activity date back more than 2,000 years (Mesulam and Perry, 1972). Until recently, however, immune functions were thought to reflect specific and nonspecific physiological responses to pathogens or tissue damage. It is now clear that the immune system is tightly regulated and integrated with the nervous and endocrine systems and that social events influence immune function through these systems. A bidirectional communication network comprised of soluble ligands and cellular receptors links both afferent and efferent functions of the immune system to the nervous and endocrine systems. Thus, a stimulus within the nervous system that activates the sympathetic adrenomedullary and HPA axis results in peripheral release of catecholamines and adrenal steroids, respectively, that have immunoregulatory potential. Similarly, a challenge within host tissue that induces an inflammatory response (e.g., an infection or a wound) results in the release of cytokines that stimulate peripheral and central circuits of the nervous system. This communication provides an important link through which the neuroendocrine response modulates the development of an inflammatory response at a site of challenge (Kusnecov et al., 1999; Maier and Watkins, 1998).

Personal ties are capable of activating aspects of innate or natural immunity that lead to the expression of illness behaviors (e.g., fever, reduced food and water intake, reduced social and sexual activity, depressed mood). These behaviors are some of the earliest responses to infectious or inflammatory challenges (Maier and Watkins, 1998). Natural immunity also encodes a number of protein molecules that provide initial resistance to the replication and spread of microbial pathogens and set the microenvironmental stage for the subsequent development of specific immune responses necessary to eliminate the pathogen (Bonneau et al., 1991). Among the protein molecules induced during challenge are the proinflammatory cytokines (e.g., IL-1, TNF, and IL-6). These cytokine responses represent peripheral signals that are conveyed through the blood-brain barrier to the central nervous system to induce illness/sickness behaviors (Fleshner et al., 1997).

Stress mediators associated with personal ties can be protective and adaptive as well as damaging. For example, significantly larger numbers of leukocytes were found in the skin of stressed animals both before and after experimental introduction of antigen (Dhabhar and McEwen, 1999), suggesting that stress prepared the immune system to respond to challenges such as infection. The bidirectional effects of stress on skin immunity are mediated by the adrenal hormones corticosterone and epinephrine. However, while acute stress is immunoenhancing, chronic stress is immunosuppressive (Dhabhar and McEwen, 1997; Dhabhar et al., 1995).

The chronic stress of caring for a relative with dementia was linked with elevated SAM and HPA activation and diminished immune function, such as reduced proliferative responses of peripheral blood leukocytes (Kiecolt-Glaser et al., 1991), lower natural killer cell response (Esterling et al., 1994), and impaired antibody response to influenza virus vaccine (Kiecolt-Glaser et al., 1996). Similar results have emerged from studies of the effects of psychosocial stress on vaccine responses. Using the stress of taking a university examination (Glaser et al., 1992) or the chronic stress of being a caregiver (Kiecolt-Glaser et al., 1996; Glaser et al., 1998), the response to vaccination was examined during the stressful period. In both cases, vaccine responses were attenuated in the stressed groups. Caregivers of relatives with progressive dementia have also shown impaired wound healing relative to controls matched for age and family income (Kiecolt-Glaser et al., 1995, 1998).

Alteration of immune function has been observed among persons in marital conflict (Kiecolt-Glaser et al., 1987). Specifically, negative or hostile behaviors during a marital conflict produce greater and/or more persistent alterations in autonomic activation and circulating stress hormones. Couples characterized by high, relative to low, negative behaviors during a marital conflict also show greater decrements over the 24 hours of study on natural killer cell lysis, the blastogenic response to two mitogens, and the proliferative response to a monoclonal antibody to the T3 receptor (Kiecolt-Glaser et al., 1994).

PERSONAL TIES AND INFECTIOUS DISEASE

In an experimental study of stress and infectious illness, healthy volunteers reported their level of stress and were exposed to saline or one of several strains of respiratory virus (Cohen et al., 1991). Following inoculation, subjects were quarantined and monitored for the development of respiratory illness. After seven days of quarantine, each participant was classified as not infected, infected but not ill, or infected and ill. No participant exposed to saline became ill, and about a third of the participants exposed to the cold viruses became ill. Results revealed that three measures of stress were related to disease onset: (1) a stressful life event scale to measure the cumulative event load, (2) a perceived-stress scale to assess perceptions of overload-induced stress, (3) and a measure of negative affect. For all three measures, participants who reported high stress were more likely to develop an infection than those who reported low stress (Cohen et al., 1991). Subsequent research has determined that risk of infection was increased most by stressors lasting over a month, especially those involving disruptions in personal ties (i.e., social conflicts, unemployment, and underemployment; Cohen et al., 1998; Glaser et al., 1999).

Social influences on infectious disease processes have also been linked with gene expression. In an experimental model of pyschosocial stress, the stress of social disruption caused by reorganizing established murine hierarchies during a respiratory viral infection significantly increased mortality compared to the stress of physical restraint in home cage control animals (Padgett and Sheridan, 1999). The increased severity of the infection leading to mortality was associated with hyper-inflammatory responses due to overexpression of key cytokine genes. Enhanced gene expression led to increased cell trafficking and accumulation in the lungs of infected animals, which in turn led to tissue consolidation and compromised lung function. These results contrasted with animals undergoing the stress of physical restraint, which is devoid of social interactions, but nonetheless activates the HPA axis in a similar fashion to the psychosocial stressor. However, hypo-inflammatory responses during respiratory viral infection were observed in these animals, due to suppression of cytokine responses by glucocorticoid hormones. Under these conditions, no increase in mortality was observed. Such findings underscore the unique significance of social interactional stressors in activating overexpression of cytokine genes implicated in increased mortality risks.

The specific nature of the personal ties, particularly their hierarchical features, also plays a major role in the individual response to stress and susceptibility to infectious disease. For example, in the social disruption paradigm described above, dominant male mice, when latently infected in the trigeminal ganglia with herpes simplex virus (HSV, a model for recurrent herpes labialis in humans), were twice as likely as subordinate animals to reactivate and shed infectious virus when their social environment was disrupted by reorganization (Padgett et al., 1998). The psychosocial nature of the stressor was also important in this model, simply stressing latently infected mice by restraint did not cause reactivation. Again, it is social interactional stress that activates physiological signals modulating the expression of individual host/pathogen genes. In the model of latent HSV infection, the inactive viral genome represents an environmental (or foreign) gene that has parasitized the host. It resides in the neurons of the trigeminal ganglia and remains latent or inactive until an appropriate set of physiological signals is received. Importantly, it is psychosocial, not general, stress that provides the appropriate signals for reactivation of the viral genes leading to recurrent infection and the shedding of infectious virus.

SOCIAL RELATIONAL ROUTES TO HEALTH

A recent review of epidemiological research shows that, in each study examined, mortality was significantly lower among persons who were more socially integrated (Berkman, 1995). Such studies are, however, limited in their ability to address questions of causality between social relationships and health (Berscheid and Reis, 1998) because a large number of factors (sociodemographic, geographic, occupational, personality) covary with measures of social integration.

Initial assessments of social isolation (or integration) emphasized objective features of social support such as the size or density of one's social network and frequency of contact with relatives and friends. Subsequent studies elaborated more subjective and/or functional aspects, such as the perception of emotional and instrumental support and assistance provided by others (Cohen, 1988; Cohen and Wills, 1985; Vaux, 1988). The social support field has been increasingly differentiated into specific substantive areas, such as the role of social support in stress and coping (Thoits, 1995), social support in family relationships (Pierce et al., 1996), social support and personality (Pierce et al., 1997), and social support in differential survival from various health challenges, such as myocardial infarction (e.g., Ruberman et al., 1984) or cancer (e.g., Spiegel et al., 1981). The latter work illustrates the "buffering model" of social support (Cohen, 1988; Cohen and Willis, 1985), which is also illustrated by research on medical students undergoing the stress of exams. Findings showed stress-induced decrements in immune functioning, but the decline was particularly pronounced for those lacking social buffers (i.e., medical students who reported being lonely; Kiecolt-Glaser et al., 1984; Glaser et al., 1992).

Other research examines possible mechanisms through which social support impacts health through behavioral routes, such as the extent to which "significant others" promote and encourage positive health practices (Berkman, 1995; Spiegel and Kimerling, in press; Taylor et al., 1997). Feeling socially embedded may enhance the salubrious effects of restorative behaviors such as sleep (Cacioppo et al., in press b). Sleep is a quintessential act of restoration that is performed without immediate social contact, indeed without much explicit awareness at all. Although lonely individuals slept as many hours per day as normal and socially embedded individuals, responses to the Pittsburgh Sleep Quality Index (PSQI) revealed that lonely individuals reported poorer sleep quality, longer sleep latency, longer perceived sleep duration, and greater daytime dysfunction due to sleepiness than socially embedded individuals (Buysse et al., 1989). Other data confirmed that lonely individuals slept less efficiently, took slightly longer to fall asleep, evidenced longer REM latency, and had more frequent micro-awakenings during the night than embedded and normal individuals (Cacioppo et al., in press b). Thus, the restorative act of sleep was more efficient and effective in socially embedded than in lonely individuals.

The most extensive research on how social ties influence health, however, pertains to the underlying physiological routes (e.g., Uchino et al., 1996; Seeman, 1996; Seeman and McEwen, 1996; Cohen and Herbert, 1996; Kang et al., 1998; Kiecolt-Glaser et al., 1994). Meta-analyses of the experimental literature support the hypothesis that perceived social isolation is associated with physiological adjustments, with the most reliable effects found for blood pressure, catecholamines, and aspects of both cellular and humoral immune function (Uchino et al., 1996; see also Seeman and McEwen, 1996). In a study of carotid atherosclerosis in middle-aged men, higher intima media thickness of the carotid artery was found in those living alone than in cohabitating counterparts even after controlling for age, health status, education level, saturated-fat consumption, and smoking (Helminen et al., 1995). Although individual differences in personality play a role, the biological effects of loneliness are evident even after controlling for common individual differences (e.g., extroversion, neuroticism) and in intervention studies designed to reduce social isolation and improve physiological functioning (Cacioppo et al., in press b; Uchino et al., 1996). People's beliefs, attitudes, and values pertaining to others appear to be especially important, because subjective indices of social isolation have been found to be more powerful predictors of stress and health than objective indices (e.g., Seeman et al., 1997; Uchino et al., 1996).

Social relationship researchers looking at attachments in early and later life and at close personal relationships, including marital and family ties, have described some features of deep, meaningful, loving human connections (Ryff and Singer, 2000). Numerous investigations have examined the nature of affect in intimate relationships, its developmental course over time, and related expressions of emotion during marital interaction (e.g., Carstensen et al., 1995, 1996; Gottman, 1994; Gottman and Levenson, 1992). Collectively, research on interpersonal flourishing gives greater attention to the emotional upside of significant social relationships and their consequences for improved health (see Ryff and Singer, 1998, 2000; Taylor et al., 2000). Of particular importance are studies that track the cumulative long-term features of social relational experience and its biological sequelae. Individuals on positive relationship pathways (positive ties with parents in childhood, intimate ties with spouse in adulthood) are less likely to show high allostatic load compared to those on negative relationship pathways, and such relational strengths also appear to offer protection against cumulative economic adversity (Singer and Ryff, 1999). Such findings call for greater understanding of the neurobiological processes that underlie positive social relationships and their role in health protection and promotion. Across these diverse areas of inquiry, longitudinal studies are also needed to help disentangle causal directionality among psychosocial and physiological factors.

RECOMMENDATIONS

NIH studies of the links between the social world and health should focus on the underlying causal (including reciprocal) mechanisms in both animals and humans. The objective is to understand interrelationships between social interaction and correlative biological phenomena.   This work should include:

- studies that explicate the links between social relationships and gene expression, brain structure and function, and neuroimmunological activity;
- investigations that identify pathways through which social ties and interacting biological systems influence health practices and behaviors;
- longitudinal studies that link cumulative social relational profiles with cumulative biological profiles (e.g., allostatic load);
- increased emphasis on the collection of biomarkers in epidemiological studies of social relationships and health;
- extensions of traditional laboratory studies to include experience sampling methodologies and corresponding ambulatory neurobiological assessments;
- multilevel integrative studies working at the interface of social interaction, emotion and brain activity, and downstream endocrinological and immunological processes.

REFERENCES

Anisman H, Zaharia MD, Meaney MJ, Merali Z. 1998 "Do early-life events permanently alter behavioral and hormonal responses to stressors?" *International Journal of Developmental Neuroscience* 16/3-4:149-164.

Baumeister RF, Leary MR. 1995 "The need to belong: Desire for interpersonal attachments as a fundamental human motivation" *Psychological Bulletin* 117/3:497-529.

Becker A. 1999 "Acculturation and Disordered Eating in Fiji" Paper presented at the annual meeting of the American Psychiatric Association, May 19, Washington DC.

Berkman LF. 1995 "The role of social relations in health promotion" *Psychosomatic Medicine* 57/3:245-254.

Berkman LF, Breslow L. 1983 *Health and Ways of Living* (New York: Oxford University Press).

Berkman LF, Syme SL. 1979 "Social networks, host resistance, and mortality: A nine-year follow-up study of Alameda County residents" *American Journal of Epidemiology* 109/2:186-204.

Berscheid E, Reis HT. 1998 "Attraction and close relationships" in Gilbert DT, Fiske ST, Lindzey G (eds.). *The Handbook of Social Psychology, Vol. 2, 4th Ed.* (Boston MA: McGraw-Hill) 193-281.

Bonneau RH, Sheridan JF, Feng NG, Glaser R. 1991 "Stress-induced effects on cell-mediated innate and adaptive mammary components of the murine immune response to herpes simplex virus infection" *Brain, Behavior, and Immunity* 5/3:274-295.

Buysse DJ, Reynolds CF, Monk TH, Berman SR, Kupfer C. 1989 "The Pittsburgh sleep quality index: A new instrument for psychiatric practice and research" *Psychiatry Research* 28:193-213.

Cacioppo JT, Berntson GG, Sheridan JF, McClintock MK. In press a. "Social neuroscience and multi-level integrative analyses of human behavior: The complementing nature of social and biological approaches" *Psychological Bulletin.*

Cacioppo JT, Ernst JM, Burleson MH, McClintock MK, Malarkey WB, Hawkley LC, Kowalewski RB, Paulsen A, Hobson JA, Hugdahl K, Spiegel D, Berntson GG. In press b. "Lonely traits and concomitant physiological processes: The MacArthur Social Neuroscience Studies" *International Journal of Psychophysiology.*

Caldji C, Tannenbaum B, Sharma S, Francis D, Plotsky PM, Meaney MJ. 1998 "Maternal care during infancy regulates the development of neural systems mediating the expression of fearfulness in the rat" *Proceedings of the National Academy of Sciences of the United States of America* 95/9:5335-5340.

Carstensen LL, Gottman JM, Levenson RW. 1995 "Emotional behavior in long-term marriage" *Psychology and Aging* 10/1:140-149.

Carstensen LL, Graff J, Levenson RW, Gottman JM. 1996 "Affect in intimate relationships: The developmental course of marriage" in Magai C, McFadden SH (eds.). *Handbook of Emotion, Adult Development, and Aging* (San Diego CA: Academic Press) 227-247.

Carter CS. 1998 "Neuroendocrine perspectives on social attachment and love" *Psychoneuroendocrinology* 23/8:779-818.

Cohen S. 1988 "Psychosocial models of the role of social support in the etiology of physical disease" *Health Psychology* 7/3:269-297.

Cohen S, Herbert TB. 1996 "Health psychology: Psychological factors and physical disease from the perspective of human psychoneuroimmunology" *Annual Review of Psychology* 47:113-142.

Cohen S, Syme SL (eds). 1985 *Social Support and Health* (Orlando FL: Academic Press).

Cohen S, Wills TA. 1985 "Stress, social support, and the buffering hypothesis" *Psychological Bulletin* 98/2:310-357.

Cohen S, Tyrrell DA, Smith AP. 1991 "Psychological stress and susceptibility to the common cold" *New England Journal of Medicine* 325/9:606-612.

Cohen S, Frank E, Doyle WJ, Skoner DP, Rabin BS, Gwaltney JM Jr. 1998 "Types of stressors that increase susceptibility to the common cold in healthy adults" *Health Psychology* 17/3:214-223.

Damasio AR. 1994 *Descartes' Error: Emotion, Reason, and the Human Brain* (New York: G.P. Putnam).

Davidson, RJ. 1998 "Affective style and affective disorders: Perspectives from affective neuroscience" *Cognition and Emotion* 12:307-330.

Davidson RJ, Rickman M. 1999 "Behavioral inhibition and the emotional circuitry of the brain: Stability and plasticity during the early childhood years" in Schmidt LA, Schulkin J (eds.). *Extreme Fear and Shyness: Origins and Outcomes* (New York: Oxford University Press).

Davidson RJ, Ekman P, Saron CD, Senulis JA, Friesen WV. 1990 "Approach-withdrawal and cerebral asymmetry: Emotional expression and brain physiology" *Journal of Personality and Social Psychology* 58/2:330-341.

Davidson RJ, Marshall JR, Tomarken AJ, Henriques JB. 2000 "While a phobic waits: Regional brain electrical and autonomic activity in social phobics during anticipation of public speaking" *Biological Psychiatry* 47/2:85-95.

Dhabhar FS, McEwen BS. 1997 "Acute stress enhances while chronic stress suppresses cell-mediated immunity in vivo: A potential role for leukocyte trafficking" *Brain, Behavior, and Immunity* 11/4:286-306.

Dhabhar FS, McEwen BS. 1999 "Enhancing versus suppressive effects of stress hormones on skin immune function" *Proceedings of the National Academy of Sciences of the United States of America* 96/3:1059-1064.

Dhabhar FS, Miller AH, McEwen BS, Spencer RL. 1995 "Effects of stress on immune cell distribution. Dynamics and hormonal mechanisms" *Journal of Immunology* 154/10:5511-5527.

Ekman P, Davidson RJ (eds.). 1994 *The Nature of Emotion: Fundamental Questions* (New York: Oxford University Press).

Ell K, Nishimoto R, Mediansky L, Mantell J, Hamovitch M. 1992 "Social relations, social support and survival among patients with cancer" *Journal of Psychosomatic Research* 36/6:531-541.

Esterling BA, Kiecolt-Glaser JK, Bodnar JC, Glaser R. 1994 "Chronic stress, social support, and persistent alterations in the natural killer cell response to cytokines in older adults" *Health Psychology* 13/4:291-298.

Ewart CK, Taylor CB, Kraemer HC, Agras WS. 1991 "High blood pressure and marital discord: Not being nasty matters more than being nice" *Health Psychology* 10/3:155-163.

Farah MJ, Wilson KD, Drain M, Tanaka JN. 1998 "What is 'special' about face perception?" *Psychological Review* 105/3:482-498.

Fleshner M, Silbert L, Deak T, Goehler LE, Martin D, Watkins LR, Maier SF. 1997 "TNF-alpha-induced corticosterone elevation but not serum protein or corticosteroid binding globulin reduction is vagally mediated" *Brain Research Bulletin* 44/6:701-706.

Friedman HS, Tucker JS, Schwartz JE, Tomlinson-Keasey C, Martin LR, Wingard DL, Criqui MH. 1995 "Psychosocial and behavioral predictors of longevity: The aging and death of the 'termites'" *American Psychologist* 50/3:69-78.

Funch DP, Marshall J. 1983 "The role of stress, social support and age in survival from breast cancer" *Journal of Psychosomatic Research* 27/1:77-83.

Ganster DC, Victor B. 1988 "The impact of social support on mental and physical health" *British Journal of Medical Psychology* 61:17-36.

Gardner WL, Gabriel S, Diekman AB. 2000 "Interpersonal processes" in Cacioppo JT, Tassinary LG, Bernston GG (eds.). *Handbook of Psychophysiology* (New York: Cambridge University Press) 643-664.

Glaser R, Kiecolt-Glaser JK, Bonneau RH, Malarkey W, Kennedy S, Hughes J. 1992 "Stress-induced modulation of the immune response to recombinant hepatitis B vaccine" *Psychosomatic Medicine* 54/1:22-29.

Glaser R, Kiecolt-Glaser JK, Malarkey WB, Sheridan JF. 1998 "The influence of psychological stress on the immune response to vaccines" *Annals of the New York Academy of Sciences* 840:649-655.

Glaser R, Rabin B, Chesney M, Cohen S, Naatelson B. 1999. "Stress-induced immunomodulation: Are there implications for infectious diseases?" *Journal of the American Medical Association* 281/24:2268-2270.

Goldin-Meadow S, Mylander C. 1983 "Gestural communication in deaf children: Noneffect of parental input on language development" *Science* 221/4608:372-374.

Goodwin JS, Hunt WC, Key CR, Samet JM. 1987 "The effect of marital status on stage, treatment, and survival of cancer patients" *Journal of the American Medical Association* 258/21:3125-3130.

Gottlieb G. 1998 "Normally occurring environmental and behavioral influences on gene activity: From central dogma to probabilistic epigenesis" *Psychological Review* 105/4:792-802.

Gottman JM. 1994 *What Predicts Divorce? The Relationship Between Marital Processes and Marital Outcomes* (Hillsdale NJ: Lawrence Erlbaum).

Gottman JM, Levenson RW. 1992 "Marital processes predictive of later dissolution: Behavior, physiology, and health" *Journal of Personality and Social Psychology* 63/2:221-233.

Helminen A, Rankinen T, Mercuri M, Rauramaa R. 1995 "Carotid atherosclerosis in middle-aged men: Relation to conjugal circumstances and social support" *Scandinavian Journal of Social Medicine* 23/13:167-172.

House JS, Landis KR, Umberson D. 1988 "Social relationships and health" *Science* 241/4865:540-545.

House JS, Lepkowski JM, Kinney AM, Mero RP, Kessler RC, Herzog AR. 1994 "The social stratification of aging and health" *Journal of Health and Social Behavior* 35/3:213-234.

Huttenlocher PR. 1990 "Morphometric study of human cerebral cortex development" *Neuropsychologia* 28/6:517-527.

Joffres M, Reed DM, Nomura AM. 1985 "Psychosocial processes and cancer incidence among Japanese men in Hawaii" *American Journal of Epidemiology* 121/14:488-500.

Kalin NH, Shelton SE, Rickman M, Davidson RJ. 1998 "Individual differences in freezing and cortisol in infant and mother rhesus monkeys" *Behavioral Neuroscience* 112/1:251-254.

Kalin NH, Shelton, SE, Davidson RJ. 2000 "Cerebrospinal fluid corticotropin releasing hormone levels are elevated in monkeys with patterns of brain activity associated with fearful temperament" *Biological Psychiatry* 47/7:579-585.

Kang DH, Coe CL, Karaszewski J, McCarthy DO. 1998 "Relationship of social support to stress responses and immune function in healthy and asthmatic adolescents" *Research in Nursing and Health* 21:117-128.

Kelley JE, Lumley MA, Leisen JC. 1997 "Health effects of emotional disclosure in rheumatoid arthritis patients" *Health Psychology* 16/4:331-340.

Kennedy S, Kiecolt-Glaser JK, Glaser R. 1988 "Immunological consequences of acute and chronic stressors: Mediating role of interpersonal relationships" *British Journal of Medical Physiology* 61:77-85.

Kiecolt-Glaser JK, Garner W, Speicher C, Penn GM, Holliday J, Glaser R. 1984 "Psychosocial modifiers of immunocompetence in medical students" *Psychosomatic Medicine* 46/1:7-14.

Kiecolt-Glaser JK, Fisher LD, Ogrocki P, Stout JC, Speicher CE, Glaser R. 1987 "Marital quality, marital disruption, and immune function" *Psychosomatic Medicine* 49/1:13-34.

Kiecolt-Glaser JK, Dura JR, Speicher CE, Trask OJ, Glaser R. 1991 "Spousal caregivers of dementia victims: Longitudinal changes in immunity and health" *Psychosomatic Medicine* 53/4:345-362.

Kiecolt-Glaser JK, Malarkey WB, Cacioppo JT, Glaser R. 1994 "Stressful personal relationships: Immune and endocrine function" in Glaser R, Kiecolt-Glaser JK (eds.). *Handbook of Human Stress and Immunity* (San Diego: Academic Press) 321-339.

Kiecolt-Glaser JK, Marucha PT, Malarkey WB, Mercado AM, Glaser R. 1995 "Slowing of wound healing by psychological stress" *Lancet* 346/8984:1194-1196.

Kiecolt-Glaser JK, Glaser R, Gravenstein S, Malarkey WB, Sheridan J. 1996 "Chronic stress alters the immune response to influenza virus vaccine in older adults" *Proceedings of the National Academy of Sciences of the United States of America* 93/7:3043-3047.

Kiecolt-Glaser JK, Glaser R, Cacioppo JT, MacCallum RC, Snydersmith M, Kim C, Malarkey WB. 1997 "Marital conflict in older adults: Endocrinological and immunological correlates" *Psychosomatic Medicine* 59/4:339-349.

Kiecolt-Glaser JK, Page GG, Marucha PT, MacCallum RC, Glaser R. 1998 "Psychological influences on surgical recovery: Perspectives from psychoneuroimmunology" *American Psychologist* 53/11:1209-1218.

Kusnecov AW, Liang R, Shurin G. 1999 "T-lymphocyte activation increases hypothalamic and amygdaloid expression of CRH mRNA and emotional reactivity to novelty" *Journal of Neuroscience* 19/11:4533-4543.

Levenson RW, Carstensen LL, Gottman JM. 1993 "Long-term marriage: Age, gender, and satisfaction" *Psychology and Aging* 8/2:301-313.

Liu D, Dioro J, Tannenbaum B, Caldji C, Francis D, Freedman A, Sharma S, Pearson D, Plotsky PM, Meaney MJ. 1997 "Maternal care, hippocampal glucocorticoid receptors, and hypothalamic-pituitary-adrenal responses to stress" *Science* 277/5332:1659-1662.

Maier SF, Watkins LR. 1998 "Cytokines for psychologists: Implications for bidirectional immune-to-brain communication for understanding behavior, mood, and cognition" *Psychological Review* 105/1:83-107.

Malarkey WB, Kiecolt-Glaser JK, Pearl D, Glaser R. 1994 "Hostile behavior during marital conflict alters pituitary and adrenal hormones" *Psychosomatic Medicine* 56/1:41-51.

Malarkey WB, Wu H, Cacioppo JT, Malarkey KL, Poehlmann KM, Claser R, Kiecolt-Glaser JK. 1996 "Chronic stress down-regulates growth hormone gene expression in peripheral blood mononuclear cells of older adults" *Endocrine* 5/1:33-39.

Manuck SB, Marsland AL, Kaplan JR, Williams JK. 1995 "The pathogenicity of behavior and its neuroendocrine mediation: An example from coronary artery disease" *Psychosomatic Medicine* 57/3:275-283.

Marangoni C, Ickes W. 1989 "Loneliness: A theoretical review with implications for measurement" *Journal of Social and Personal Relationships* 6/1:93-128.

Meaney MJ, Sapolsky RM, McEwen BS. 1985 "The development of the glucocorticoid receptor system in the rat limbic brain. II. An autoradiographic study" *Brain Research* 350/1-2:165-168.

Meaney MJ, Bhatnagar S, Larocque S, McCormick CM, Shanks N, Sharma S, Smythe J, Viau V, Plotsky PM. 1996 "Early environment and the development of individual differences in the hypothalamic-pituitary-adrenal stress response" in Pfeffer CR (ed.). *Severe Stress and Mental Disturbance in Children* (Washington DC: American Psychiatric Association Press) 85-127.

Mesulam MM, Perry J. 1972 "The diagnosis of love-sickness: Experimental psychophysiology without the polygraph" *Psychophysiology* 9/5:546-551.

Myers DG, Diener E. 1995 "Who is happy?" *Psychological Science* 6/1:10-19.

Padgett DA, Sheridan JF. 1999 "Social stress, dominance, and increased mortality from an influenza viral infection" (Unpublished paper, Department of Oral Biology, Ohio State University, Columbus, OH).

Padgett DA, Sheridan JF, Dorne J, Berntson GG, Candelora J, Glaser R. 1998 "Social stress and the reactivation of latent herpes simplex virus type 1" *Proceedings of the National Academy of Sciences of the United States of America* 12:7231-7235.

Panksepp J. 1998 *Affective Neuroscience: The Foundations of Human and Animal Emotions* (New York: Oxford University Press).

Pescosolido B. 1986 "Migration, medical care and the lay referral system: A network theory of adult socialization" *American Journal of Sociology* 51:523-590.

Pescosolido B. 1991 "Illness careers and network ties: A conceptual model of utilization and compliance" *Advances in Medical Sociology* 2:161-184.

Petersson M, Alster P, Lundeberg T, Uvnäs-Moberg K. 1996 "Oxytocin causes long-term decrease of blood pressure in female and male rats" *Physiology and Behavior* 60:1311-1315.

Pierce GR, Sarason BR, Sarason IG. 1996 *Handbook of Social Support and the Family* (New York: Plenum).

Pierce GR, Lakey B, Sarason IG, Sarason BR. 1997 *Sourcebook of Social Support and Personality* (New York: Plenum).

Pinker S. 1997 *How the Mind Works* (New York: Norton).

Rauch SL, Savage CR, Alpert NM, Fischman AJ, Jenike MA. 1997 "The functional neuroanatomy of anxiety: A study of three disorders using positron emission tomography and symptom provocation" *Biological Psychiatry* 42/6:446-452.

Reis HT. In press "Relationships, experiences, and emotional well-being" in Ryff CD, Singer B (eds.). *Emotion, Social Relationships, and Health* (New York: Oxford University Press).

Repetti RL, Taylor SE, Seeman TE. In press "Risky families: Family social environments and the mental and physical health of offspring" *Psychological Bulletin.*

Reynolds P, Kaplan GA. 1990 "Social connections and risk for cancer: Prospective evidence from the Alameda County Study" *Behavioral Medicine* 16/3:101-110.

Rodin J. 1986 *Health, Control and Aging* (Hillsdale NJ: Earlbaum).

Ruberman W, Weinblatt E, Goldberg JD, Chaudhary BS. 1984 "Psychosocial influences on mortality after myocardial infarction" *New England Journal of Medicine* 311/9:552-559.

Ryff CD, Singer B. 1998 "The contours of positive human health" *Psychological Inquiry 9/1:1-28.

Ryff CD, Singer B. 2000. "Interpersonal flourishing: A positive health agenda for the new millennium" *Personality and Social Psychology Review* 4:30-44.

Seeman TE. 1996 "Social ties and health: The benefits of social integration" *Annals of Epidemiology* 6/5:442-451.

Seeman TE, Berkman LF, Kohout F, Lacroix A, Glynn R, Blazer D. 1993 "Intercommunity variation in the association between social ties and mortality in the elderly: A comparative analysis of three communities" *Annals of Epidemiology* 3:325-335.

Seeman TE, McEwen BS. 1996 "Impact of social environment characteristics on neuroendocrine regulation" *Psychosomatic Medicine* 58/5:459-471.

Seeman TE, Singer BH, Rowe JW, Horwitz RI, McEwen BS. 1997 "Price of adaptation—Allostatic load and its health consequences" *Archives of Internal Medicine* 157/19:2259-2268.

Singer B, Ryff CD. 1999 "Hierarchies of life histories and health risk" *Annals of the New York Academy of Sciences* 869:96-115.

Skantze HB, Kaplan J, Pettersson K, Manuck S, Blomqvist N, Kyes R, Williams K, Bondjers G. 1998 "Psychosocial stress causes endothelial injury in cynomolgus monkeys via beta1-adrenoceptor activation" *Atherosclerosis* 136/1:153-161.

Spiegel D, Bloom JR, Yalom I. 1981 "Group support for patients with metastatic cancer: A randomized outcome study" *Archives of General Psychiatry* 38:527-533.

Spiegel D, Kimerling R. In press "Group psychotherapy for women with breast cancer: Relationships among social support, emotional expression, and survival" in Ryff CD, Singer B (eds.). *Emotion, Social Relationships, and Health* (New York: Oxford University Press).

Sternberg RJ, Hojjat M (eds.). 1997 *Satisfaction in Close Relationships* (New York: Guilford).

Suomi S. 1999 "Jumpy monkeys" Invited address presented at the annual meeting of the American Psychological Society, 4 June, Denver CO.

Taylor SE, Repetti RL, Seeman T. 1997 "Health psychology: What is an unhealthy environment and how does it get under the skin?" *Annual Review of Psychology* 48:411-447.

Taylor SE, Kemeny ME, Reed GM, Bower JE, Gruenewald TL. 2000. "Psychological resources, positive illusions, and health" *American Psychologist* 55/1:99-109.

Thoits PA. 1995 "Stress, coping, and social support processes: Where are we? What next?" *Journal of Health and Social Behavior* Spec No:53-79.

Uehara E. 1990 "Dual exchange theory, social networks, and informal social support" *American Journal of Sociology* 96/3:521-557.

Uchino BN, Cacioppo JT, Kiecolt-Glaser JK. 1996 "The relationship between social support and physiological processes: A review with emphasis on underlying mechanisms and implications for health" *Psychological Bulletin* 119/3:488-531.

Uvnäs-Moberg K. 1997 "Physiological and endocrine effects of social contact" *Annals of the New York Academy of Sciences* 807:146-163.

Uvnäs-Moberg K. 1998 "Oxytocin may mediate the benefits of positive social interaction and emotions" *Psychoneuroendocrinology* 23:819-835.

Vaux A. 1988 *Social Support: Theory, Research, and Intervention* (New York: Praeger).

Wu H, Wang J, Cacioppo JT, Glaser R, Kiecolt-Glaser JK, Malarkey WB. 1999 "Chronic stress associated with spousal caregiving of patients with Alzheimer's dementia is associated with downregulation of B-lymphocyte GH mRNA" *Journals of Gerontology. Series A, Biological Sciences and Medical Sciences* 54/4:M212-M215.

6

Collective Properties and Healthy Communities

The previous chapter demonstrated the strong connection between personal ties and a variety of health outcomes. A large body of research also documents the association of health-related outcomes with the socioeconomic characteristics of community contexts. For example, the ecological concentration of poverty correlates to infant mortality, low birth weight, child maltreatment, and adolescent violence as well as depression, homicide, victimization, cardiovascular diseases, and all-cause mortality. At the other end of the spectrum, communities with high socioeconomic status appear to promote health in both children and adults. Research indicates that risk and protective factors in the community environment are not solely attributable to individual-level attributes or behavioral lifestyles. Moreover, predisease pathways in individuals may interact with community characteristics in ways that alter the risk for disease.

In this chapter we therefore highlight the collective properties of social environments, alongside rather than in opposition to individual factors and personal ties. Such a focus treats community contexts as important units of analysis in their own right, calling for new measurement strategies as well as methodological frameworks that do not simply treat the social context as a "trait" of the individual. Understanding the causes of variation in collective processes associated with healthy communities may provide opportunities for preventive intervention at lower cost than traditional strategies.

COMMUNITY CONTEXTS AND MULTILEVEL RESEARCH

Social characteristics vary systematically across communities along dimensions of socioeconomic status (e.g., poverty, wealth, occupational attainment), cultural context (e.g., normative guidelines), family structure and life cycle (e.g., female-headed households, child density), residential stability (e.g., home ownership and tenure), and racial/ethnic composition (e.g., racial segregation). A long history of research shows that health-related problems also vary systematically by community, often in conjunction with socioeconomic characteristics (Yen and Syme, 1999). As far back as the 1920s, urban neighborhoods characterized by poverty, residential instability, and dilapidated housing were found to suffer disproportionately higher rates of infant mortality, crime, mental illness, low birth weight, tuberculosis, physical abuse, and other factors detrimental to health (see e.g., Shaw and McKay, 1942).

This general empirical finding continues to the present day, as illustrated by the ecological "comorbidity" or spatial clustering of homicide, infant mortality, low birth weight, accidental injury, and suicide. In the period 1995-1996, for example, data from the city of Chicago reveal that census tracts with high homicide rates tend to be spatially contiguous to other tracts high in homicide. Perhaps more interesting, more than 75 percent of such tracts also contain a high level of clustering for low birth weight and infant mortality and more than 50 percent for accidental injuries (Sampson, forthcoming). Suicide is more distinct, although even here the spatial clustering is significant. The ecological concentration of homicide, low birth weight, infant mortality, and injury indicates that there may be geographic "hot spots" for unhealthy outcomes.

Not only do social characteristics vary systematically with health across communities, a growing body of contextually oriented research has linked community social characteristics with variations in individual-level health. Simply put, even when individual attributes and behaviors are taken into account, there is evidence of direct risk factors linked to environmental context (Robert, 1999a). Recent analyses of the longitudinal Alameda County Health study in northern California, for example, found that self-reported fair/poor health was 70 percent higher for residents of concentrated poverty areas than for residents of nonpoverty areas, independent of age, sex, income, education, smoking status, body mass index, and alcohol consumption (Yen and Kaplan, 1999a). In a related study, the age and sex-adjusted odds for mortality were more than 50 percent higher (odds ratio = 1.58) for residents in areas characterized by poverty and deteriorated housing, after adjusting for income, race/ethnicity, smoking, body mass index, alcohol consumption, and perceived health status (Yen and Kaplan, 1999b). Such patterns are not limited to the United States. A multilevel study in

Sweden found a similar elevated risk of poor health for residents of lower socioeconomic status communities, controlling for age, sex, education, body mass index, smoking, and physical activity (Malmstrom et al., 1999).

EXPERIMENTAL EVIDENCE

Correlational and observational studies suffer well-known weaknesses with respect to making causal inferences. It may be, for example, that individuals with poor health selectively migrate to or are left behind in poor neighborhoods. In the case of individual selection, the correlation of health with community characteristics may be spurious. Experimental and quasi-experimental studies have thus begun to explore community-level effects on health outcomes. One such example is found in the Moving to Opportunity (MTO) program, a series of housing experiments in five cities that randomly assigned housing project residents to one of three groups: an experimental group receiving housing subsidies to move into low-poverty neighborhoods, a group receiving conventional (Section 8) housing assistance, and a control group receiving no special assistance. A study from the Boston MTO site showed that children of mothers in the experimental group had significantly lower prevalence of injuries, asthma attacks, and personal victimization during follow-up. The move to low-poverty neighborhoods also resulted in significant improvements in the general health status and mental health of household heads (Katz et al., 1999). Because the experimental design was used to control individual-level risk factors, a reasonable inference from these studies is that an improvement in community socioeconomic environment leads to better health and behavioral outcomes.

In short, research in social and behavioral science has established a reasonably consistent set of findings relevant to the community context of health:

• There is considerable inequality between neighborhoods and local communities along multiple dimensions of socioeconomic status.
• A number of health problems tend to cluster together at the neighborhood and larger community levels, including but not limited to violence, low birth weight, infant mortality, child maltreatment, and the risk of premature adult death.
• These two phenomena are themselves related; community-level predictors common to many health-related outcomes include concentrated poverty and/or affluence, racial segregation, family disruption, residential instability, and poor-quality housing.
• The ecological differentiation of U.S. society by factors such as social class, cultural background, race, and health (see also Chapter 7) is a

robust and apparently increasing occurrence that emerges at multiple levels of geography, whether neighborhoods, local community areas, or even states.

• The relationship between concentrated poverty and many health outcomes, especially all-cause mortality, depression, and violence, maintains when controls are introduced for individual-level risk factors. Thus, there appears to be a direct association between the social environment and health, an emerging pattern in experimental studies as well.

MECHANISMS

Taken together, these findings yield a potentially important clue in thinking about why it is that communities and larger collectivities might matter for health. If multiple and seemingly disparate health outcomes are linked together empirically across communities and are predicted by similar characteristics, there may be common underlying causes or mediating mechanisms. In particular, if "neighborhood effects" of concentrated poverty on health exist, presumably they stem from social processes that involve collective aspects of neighborhood life, such as social cohesion, spatial diffusion, local support networks, informal social control, and subcultures of violence. Yet we know little about these and other social mechanisms, especially how to measure them at the community level (Mayer and Jencks, 1989; Sampson et al., 1999). Questions about collective properties and mediating social processes pertain equally to observational and experimental studies. For example, what accounts for the apparent improved health among public-housing residents in the Boston MTO experimental group: level of safety, housing quality, social support? Establishing an effect of the environment on health is not tantamount to explaining its biological pathways or its collective-level sources.

An emerging body of research has therefore begun to explore how social processes such as mutual trust among community residents, shared expectations, density of acquaintanceship, reciprocated exchange of information, social control of public spaces, institutional resources, local support networks, and participation in voluntary associations bear on public health outcomes. For example, an index combining informal social control and social cohesion (labeled "collective efficacy") has been shown to predict rates of violence across more than 300 Chicago neighborhoods. Collective efficacy showed a strong negative relationship with the rate of neighborhood violence, after controlling for poverty, residential stability, immigrant concentration, and a set of individual-level characteristics such as age, sex, socioeconomic status, race/ethnicity and home ownership (Sampson et al., 1997). This finding held up after adjusting for prior levels of neighborhood violence that may have depressed later collective efficacy because of fear; in this model, a two-standard-deviation elevation in collective efficacy was associated with a 26 percent reduction in the expected homicide rate (Sampson et al., 1997:922). Measures of social cohesion and trust have also been found to predict mortality rates at the state level. The level of distrust (the proportion of residents in each state agreeing that most people cannot be trusted) was strongly correlated in one study (Kawachi et al., 1997) with the age-adjusted mortality rate ($r = .79$, $p < .001$). Lower levels of trust were associated with higher rates of most major causes of death, including coronary heart disease, unintentional injury, and cerebrovascular disease. A one-standard-deviation increase in trust was associated with a 9 percent lower level of mortality.

METHODOLOGICAL CHALLENGES AND RESEARCH PRIORITIES

Despite promising leads from existing research, numerous limitations must be addressed if scientific knowledge is to progress. Indeed, methodological issues such as the differential selection of individuals into communities (compositional and selection effects), indirect environmental effects that work through family and peer mechanisms, measurement error, spatial interdependence (e.g., diffusion processes), and simultaneity bias (e.g., poor health causing poverty) represent serious challenges to our ability to draw definitive conclusions on the role of neighborhood and community social contexts. Equally important, there is a need to further develop multilevel methodologies for contextually based research. Health data collected at nested levels of aggregation (e.g., neighborhood, city, state) pose important challenges to the standard analytic procedures used by health researchers. A methodological program of research is thus needed to develop tools for the proper evaluation and analysis of community-level data.

A central challenge in this regard is to build strategies for direct measurement of the social mechanisms and collective properties hypothesized to predict health. As interest in the social sciences turns increasingly to an integrated scientific approach that emphasizes individual factors in social context, a mismatch has arisen in the quality of measures (Raudenbush and Sampson, 1999). Standing behind individual measurements are decades of psychometric and biological research, producing measures that often have excellent statistical properties. In contrast, much less is known about measures of ecological settings. Neighborhood-level research in particular is dominated by the study of poverty and other demographic characteristics drawn from census data or other government statistics that do not provide information on the collective properties of administrative units. We thus recommend a concerted methodological effort to enhance the science of ecological assessment ("ecometrics") of social environments relevant to health. A major component of ecometrics is the development of systematic procedures for directly measuring community social processes, such as in population-based health surveys and systematic social observation of community environments (Sampson et al., 1999; Raudenbush and Sampson, 1999). The latter approach has used videotaping techniques to capture aspects of microcommunity environments (such as street blocks) that bear on health risks (e.g., garbage in the streets, public intoxication, unsafe housing).

A potentially fruitful direction for the National Institutes of Health (NIH) would be to support the systematic collection of benchmark data on social environments that can be compared across communities. An exemplar that might be used as a framework on which to build is the Sustainable Seattle project (Sustainable Seattle, 1999), where some 40 indicators have been collected for use as a benchmark to gauge the progress of Seattle in meeting various goals of public and civic health. An innovative combination of archival records, census data, and surveys characterizes sustainability trends across five basic areas: environment (e.g., air quality), population and resources (e.g., fuel consumption), economy (e.g., housing affordability, poverty), youth and education (e.g., high school graduation, literacy), and community health (e.g., low birth weight, neighborliness). The Leaders Roundtable in Portland, Oregon, has undertaken a similarly ambitious initiative (The Caring Community) that collects data on community health using a combination of focus groups, surveys, key stakeholder interviews, and document reviews (Green, 1999). If agreed measurement standards at the national level could be developed under NIH leadership, communities could use benchmark data to develop early warning signs with respect to changes in the quality of health environments. Ultimately, understanding the dynamics of change in communities themselves and not just the aggregated characteristics of individuals is important for establishing the sources and effects of collective properties that bear on health, in addition to effective policy responses.

In promoting efforts to reach these goals, the institutes are well positioned to take advantage of recent developments that augur well for analytic advances in the behavioral and social sciences. One is the "quasi-experimental" changes now underway across many American cities in public housing, such as the Moving to Opportunity experiments (Katz et al., 1999), voucher programs, and dispersion of concentrated poverty. By integrating econometric strategies for collecting theoretically relevant data on the collective properties of social environments with the random assignment of individuals to new social contexts, researchers are in a better position to sort out selection mechanisms and social causation mechanisms in health outcomes. We thus recommend that NIH support creative efforts to analytically exploit the planned changes that are unfolding in the public housing arena. A second window of opportunity can be found in new technologies for the mapping and identification of environmental "hot spots." Geographic information systems (GISs) exploit technological advances in ways that are transforming how research is being conducted in the social sciences. For instance, data on health outcomes can now be linked virtually in real time to address-level data bases on employment, density of liquor stores, mixed land use, and building code violations. A principal advantage of GISs is community profiling and the ability to overlay multiple health-related phenomena (e.g., deaths, cancer clusters, and accident hot spots) in time and space.

INTERACTIONS OF INDIVIDUAL AND COLLECTIVE PROPERTIES

Previous sections of this report discussed the importance of predisease pathways, but there is little research on how such pathways interact with community, environmental, and cultural contexts. Research on the collective properties of healthy communities thus needs to be integrated with the vigorous body of research on individual pathways. For example, do allostatic loads build up faster and in more destructive ways for racial/ethnic or cultural minorities living in some contexts than others? What are these environments? What mechanisms explain person-environment interactions? Are there threshold effects or leveling effects of the environment on disease risk such that individual factors become overwhelmed? What are these thresholds and for what aspects of the environment? As one example, there is evidence that race and income are not significant predictors of disease in areas of concentrated disadvantage (Yen and Syme, 1999). Multilevel studies share a unifying theme in stressing the interaction of individuals and context. Unfortunately, research has yet to systematically link validated measures of community context with the developmental course of predisease pathways and individual-level health outcomes. Although in its infancy, we believe that the multilevel study of developmental and community processes related to health is a crucial research frontier that deserves priority.

OTHER SOCIAL CONTEXTS

To be sure, health environments are not limited to geographical communities. As described elsewhere in this report, families, workplaces, religious institutions, and peer groups generate their own collective properties that bear on health. Many of these factors are in turn influenced by cultural context and background. Nonetheless, strong friendship ties and family social support networks have been found to promote individual health (Berkman and Syme, 1979). Nor are the relevant health environments limited to urban settings and areas of disadvantage. Most of the U.S. population lives in suburban areas, and the relationship of socioeconomic status and health holds at the upper end of the socioeconomic distribution as well as the lower end (Robert, 1999b). Yet much of the extant research literature is limited to the study of poverty in inner-city communities, underscoring the need to assess suburban and rural contexts. Moreover, there is a need for research on how public policies (e.g., on housing, transportation, and economic development) influence the collective properties of environments. Understanding community social processes requires a simultaneous focus on multiple social contexts and institutional (including governmental) domains.

RECOMMENDATIONS

We recommend a coordinated effort in the institutes to investigate the collective properties of social environments that extant research suggests are promising for a deeper understanding of the etiology of health outcomes and for the development of community-based prevention strategies. Because community contexts are important units of analysis in their own right, they call for concrete strategies that have heretofore been neglected in the institutes. We also underscore the importance of attending to cultural diversity in how healthy communities are defined and realized. Regarding the future, NIH-supported research on healthy communities should include the following kinds of work:

• development of a "benchmark" assessment (standardized approach) of the collective health of communities;
• selection of and support for longitudinal studies that target data augmentation and multilevel analysis, with a particular focus on person-environment interactions;
• investigation of contextual factors (e.g., cohesion, informal social control, physical disorder, local support networks) as mediators of health or disease outcomes;
• design of prevention strategies to promote aggregate-level health by changing social and community environments (e.g., regulation of smoking in public places, taxation policies).

REFERENCES

Berkman LF, Syme SL. 1979 "Social networks, host resistance, and mortality: A nine-year follow-up study of Alameda County residents" *American Journal of Epidemiology* 109/2:186-204.
Green B. 1999 *An Evaluation of the Caring Community Initiative of the Leaders Roundtable* (Portland OR: Northwest Professional Consortium, Inc.)

Katz L, Kling J, Liebman J. 1999 "Moving to opportunity in Boston: Early impacts of a housing mobility program" Paper presented at the conference "Neighborhood Effects on Low Income Families," Joint Center for Poverty Research, Northwestern University/ University of Chicago, Chicago IL, September.

Kawachi I, Kennedy BP, Lochner K, Prothrow-Stith D. 1997 "Social capital, income inequality, and mortality" *American Journal of Public Health* 87/9:1491-1498.

Malmstrom M, Sundquist J, Johansson SE. 1999 "Neighborhood environment and self-reported health status: A multilevel analysis" *American Journal of Public Health* 89/8:1181-1186.

Mayer SE, Jencks C. 1989 "Growing up in poor neighborhoods: How much does it matter?" *Science* 243/4897:1441-1445.

Raudenbush SW, Sampson RJ. 1999 "'Ecometrics': Toward a science of assessing ecological settings, with application to the systematic social observation of neighborhoods" *Sociological Methodology* 29:1-41.

Robert SA. 1999a "Neighborhood socioeconomic context and adult health. The mediating role of individual health behaviors and psychosocial factors" *Annals of the New York Academy of Sciences* 896:465-468.

Robert SA. 1999b "Socioeconomic position and health: The independent contribution of community socioeconomic context" *Annual Review of Sociology* 25:489-516.

Sampson RJ. Forthcoming "How do communities undergird or undermine human development? Relevant contexts and social mechanisms" in Booth A and Crouter AC (eds), *Does It Take a Village? Community Effects on Children, Adolescents, and Families* (Mahwah NJ: Lawrence Erlbaum).

Sampson RJ, Raudenbush SW, Earls F. 1997 "Neighborhoods and violent crime: A multilevel study of collective efficacy" *Science* 277/5328:918-924.

Sampson RJ, Morenoff JD, Earls F. 1999 "Beyond social capital: Spatial dynamics of collective efficacy for children." *American Sociological Review* 64/5:633-660.

Shaw CR, McKay HD. 1942 *Juvenile Delinquency and Urban Areas, A Study of Rates of Delinquents in Relation to Differential Characteristics of Local Communities in American Cities* (Chicago: University of Chicago Press).

Sustainable Seattle. 1999 *Indicators of a Sustainable Community: A Status Report on Long-Term Cultural, Economic, and Environmental Health for Seattle/King County* (Seattle: Sustainable Seattle).

Yen IH, Kaplan GA. 1999a "Poverty area residence and changes in depression and perceived health status: Evidence from the Alameda County Study" *International Journal of Epidemiology* 28/1:90-94.

Yen IH, Kaplan GA. 1999b "Neighborhood social environment and risk of death: Multilevel evidence from the Alameda County study" *American Journal of Epidemiology* 149/10:898-907.

Yen IH, Syme SL. 1999 "The social environment and health: A discussion of the epidemiologic literature" *Annual Review of Public Health* 20:287-308.

7

The Influence of Inequality
on Health Outcomes

Health and wealth have always been closely related (Wilkinson, 1994), and economically disadvantaged racial/ethnic minority populations in the United States experience worse health status on multiple indicators of physical health (Williams, in press). The existence of inequality—a property of the population in question—thus has important consequences for the health of individuals and groups. Better understanding of the mechanisms involved may suggest concrete ways to improve the health of both individuals and population subgroups.

SOCIOECONOMIC STATUS AND HEALTH

Health is related to both the quantitative and qualitative aspects of material and social change. Social environments that are less divisive, less undermining of self-confidence, less productive of social antagonism, and more supportive of developing skills and abilities are likely to contribute to the overall health and welfare of the population.

Socioeconomic Factors Influencing Health

An extensive literature, dating back more than a century (Sorokin, 1927; Antonovsky, 1967; Bunker et al., 1989; Williams, 1990) documents inverse associations between position in socioeconomic hierarchies and morbidity and mortality. These hierarchies have usually been defined by household income, years of education, and occupational prestige or grade.

In both industrialized and less industrialized countries, persons of higher socioeconomic status (SES) live longer and have lower rates of most diseases than their less favored counterparts (Behm, 1980; Grosse and Auffrey, 1989; Holzer et al., 1986; Department of Health and Social Security, 1980). Some studies from less industrialized countries, such as a study of Nigerian civil servants (Markovic et al., 1998), have found a positive association between SES and chronic disease. This may reflect differences in the historical time period across societies in the secular distribution of disease. In the United States, for example, higher position in the SES hierarchy was associated with greater prevalence of heart disease earlier this century, but SES is currently inversely related to cardiovascular risk (Morgenstern, 1980). Thus, apparently discrepant findings highlight the importance of attending to broader social and historical contexts.

Of particular importance is a gradient in the relationship between SES and health: each level of the hierarchy exhibits less morbidity and mortality than lower levels (Adler et al., 1994, 1999; Marmot et al., 1991). Most of the evidence supporting this relationship derives from European and North American populations, where the data are consistent and robust. At the same time, several studies document that the gradient is nonetheless characterized by a threshold, usually around the median for income, where additional increases in SES have a diminished effect in reducing morbidity and mortality rates (Kitagawa and Hauser, 1973; Pappas et al., 1993; McDonough et al., 1997; Wilkinson, 1986). Research is needed to provide greater understanding of the conditions under which particular markers of SES manifest patterns of linear or nonlinear associations with health status. We need to identify the thresholds after which weaker SES effects are observed and to characterize the social, psychological, and material risks and resources that are associated with each level of the SES hierarchy.

A growing body of research also reveals that even though overall mortality rates have been declining, socioeconomic differentials in mortality have been widening in recent decades. Comparing data from the 1960s to those for the late 1970s and 1980s, U.S. studies reveal that income and educational differentials have widened over time (Duleep, 1989; Pappas et al., 1993; Feldman et al., 1989). Similarly, widening socioeconomic differentials in mortality have been observed in England, Wales, France, Finland, Norway, and the Netherlands (Department of Health and Social Security, 1980; Kunst and Mackenbach, 1994; Mackenbach et al., 1989). Widening health disparities appear to be primarily driven by larger improvements in the health of high-SES groups compared to their lower-SES counterparts. For some health conditions, however, there has been no change in health or worsening health status over time for economically disadvantaged populations (Williams and Collins, 1995). Although differences between SES groups in access, utilization, and the quality of medical care probably play some role in the widening health inequality (Makenbach et al., 1989), increases in income and wealth inequality in both the United States and Western Europe (Danziger and Gottschalk, 1993) appear to be the driving force behind the widening health disparities (Williams and Collins, 1995).

A high degree of inequality in a given location (e.g., country, state, county, district, city) may itself be a health hazard. The countries with the smallest spread of incomes and the smallest proportion of the population in relative poverty have the longest life expectancies (Wilkinson, 1994). Evidence from multiple sources suggests that the greater the concentration of income at the upper end of the income distribution, the higher the mortality and morbidity rates (Wilkinson, 1994; Kaplan et al., 1996; Lynch et al., 1998). Socioeconomic inequality also affects health in more complicated ways. It is widely recognized that at the aggregate level average health is negatively correlated to the degree of income inequality. However, if health status depends not on absolute income but on income relative to that of some reference group, then the relationship between income and health is determined by the relative size of within-group and between-group inequality (Deaton, 1999). When the ratio of between-group to within-group inequality changes, the mix of high- and low-income status in any particular group changes. This change alters the measure of the relationship between health and income. Existing community-level evidence about socioeconomic inequality and its relationship to health implies the need for more detailed inquiries into appropriate measures of inequality.

There is considerable variation in health outcomes at all levels of socioeconomic hierarchies. Of particular importance, health outcome variance is greater at the bottom of these hierarchies—for low levels of education and income—than at the upper end. The fact that some persons low in these hierarchies have unexpectedly positive health outcomes (compared to the norm for their level) calls for future inquiry regarding the psychological, social, behavioral, and biological factors that confer protection for some individuals at the low end of the socioeconomic hierarchy.

Cumulative Pathways to Illness or Health

The provision of defensible explanations for associations between position in socioeconomic hierarchies and morbidity and mortality requires integrated investigation of psychosocial and physiological interrelationships over the life course. Most studies attempting to identify stressful life experiences and other features that predict later disease and mortality have incorporated neither long-term processes nor cumulative experience. There is a singular lack of studies integrating community-level and individual-level behavioral influences with parallel physiological dynamics to identify multilevel pathways to diverse health outcomes. Evidence does suggest that cumulative processes across multiple life domains at the individual and community levels are of central importance for understanding the relationship between SES and health (Singer and Ryff, 1999; Ryff and Singer, 2000).

Studies of income dynamics and its connection to health over the life course points to the importance of economic inequality resulting from cumulative processes, particularly permanent income (Lynch et al., 1997a, b; Felitti et al., 1998). For example, elevated permanent income, rather than current income level, shows a strong protective effect on mortality over time (Deaton, 1999). The cumulative negative impact of persistent poverty on health has also received considerable attention (Korenman and Miller, 1997). The bidirectional relationships between health and both income and wealth suggest the need for more extensive investigation of the role of permanent and transitory changes in income and unemployment on health risks (see Smith, 1999).

The import of cumulative effects also holds for psychosocial experiences. It has long been argued that early life conditions, including the fetal environment, are linked with later life expectancy and disease risks (Elo and Preston, 1992; Barker et al., 1989). However, there is great plasticity in factors influencing later-life health and length of life, and cumulative adversity and advantage are consequential. Studies of social stress and its consequences for mental health frequently also evaluate childhood and lifetime traumas as well as track chronic, enduring conditions (Singer et al., 1998). This is illustrated by results showing that a single stressor or no stressor at all produced a 1 percent increment in psychiatric disorders in children (Garmezy, 1993a, b). Two stressors in the family complex provide a 5 percent rise in the disorder rate; three stressors a 6 percent increment, and four or more stressors a 21 percent increment in the rate of childhood psychiatric disorders. Cumulatively, the presence of stressors accounted for a 33 percent rise in the disorder rate, with multiple stressors accounting for the largest proportion of the disorders.

Early life disadvantage and adversity need not lead to later negative outcomes, however, provided there are compensating positive experiences in the intervening years. Recent animal studies provide dramatic evidence that genetic predisposition can be overcome by exposure to particular environmental conditions in infancy and later life (Francis et al., 1999; Caldji et al., 1998; Liu et al., 1997). Rat pups reared in impoverished environments have greater physiological reactions to stress throughout their lives than rats reared in enriched environments (Lui et al., 1997). The effect, however, is reversible. Rats exposed to inadequate nurturing in early infancy can, if subsequently reared by a high-licking and -grooming foster mother, exhibit normal responses and healthy adult lives (Francis et al., 1999; see Chapter 4).

Recovery from and Resilience to Adversity

Equally important is clarification of mechanisms of recovery from and resistance to adversity. It is important to give equal consideration to positive aspects of people's lives and particularly to accumulation of advantage. The components leading to cumulative advantage may come in the form of starting resources (e.g., growing up in an intact family), personal capacities and abilities (e.g., intelligence, coping strategies), positive behavioral practices (e.g., exercise, proper diet), the realization of expected life transitions (e.g., job promotions, marriage), or having positive evaluations of one's life (e.g., job satisfaction, marital quality, and positive personal relationships with children, siblings, and friends).

Simultaneous consideration of cumulative adversity and advantage as they pertain to understanding health outcomes, including resilience, has been the theme of several recent investigations (Ryff et al., 1998). In understanding pathways into and recovery from episodes of depression, for example, the cumulative processes of both negative and positive valence must be identified (Singer et al., 1998). The basic point is that pathways to diverse health outcomes depend on an interplay of both positive and negative experiences across multiple life domains. (See also Chapter 3.)

At the level of physiology, an indicator of the long-term physiological response to stress conceptualized as allostatic load (McEwen, 1998; McEwen and Stellar, 1993) provides the important beginnings of a bridge between measures of cumulative psychosocial adversity relative to advantage and their biological signature. The conceptualization and measurement of this construct are described in detail in Chapter 2. Representing an index of risk across multiple physiological systems, allostatic load has been found to predict later-life incident cardiovascular disease, decline in physical and cognitive functioning, and mortality (Seeman et al., 1997). Allostatic load also represents a physiological signature of cumulative adversity relative to advantage in the domains of economic resources and social relationship (Singer and Ryff, 1999). An important research topic for the future is further investigation of linkages between cumulative SES-related adversity and cumulative physiological risk, represented by allostatic load, as well as assessment of psychosocial and behavioral factors that can offset the accumulation of such load.

The Need for Integrative Longitudinal Studies

There are few longitudinal data sets that both cover long stretches of lives (e.g., 35 plus years) and include both psychosocial and physiological risk factors as well as health outcomes. National surveys of the birth cohorts of 1946 and 1958 in England (Power and Matthews, 1997; Wadsworth and Kuh, 1997) represent valuable sources of psychosocial evidence for specification of pathways that combine sources of cumulative adversity and advantage over time. Both data sets show evidence of negative mental health consequences in adolescence and adulthood that accrue from adverse experience in early childhood as well as the influence of cumulative experience from early childhood on self-reported midlife physical health. Until recently, direct physiological assessments of these populations had not been made. With planned future longitudinal follow-up on both psychosocial and physiological indicators, the British birth cohorts represent promising sources of data for constructing integrative life history accounts of cross-time associations between socioeconomic standing and health.

In the United States, the Wisconsin Longitudinal Study (WLS; Hauser et al., 1993), which is focused on the birth cohort of 1939, is the closest to the British birth cohorts in richness of psychosocial information but goes well beyond the British studies with its in-depth assessments of educational attainment and occupational experience as well as accompanying data from siblings, spouses, and parents. WLS is, however, a random sample of the high school graduating class of 1957 in the state of Wisconsin and lacks the in-depth psychosocial assessments of infancy and early childhood found in the British birth cohorts. WLS also does not include the lowest level of the education hierarchy. Nonetheless, the age 52-53 round of WLS data collection initiated extensive inquiry on physical health and psychological well-being, and a subsample ($N = 115$) of respondents was resurveyed at age 59, at which time extensive physiological assessments were also obtained. These data have afforded an evidential basis for linking cumulative economic and relational adversity to high allostatic load (Singer and Ryff, 1999). WLS and the British birth cohorts represent the best of what is currently available on psychosocial experience across multiple life domains through time. Other important longitudinal resources, although more restricted in length of follow-up and/or coverage of psychosocial experience, are the Alameda County Study (Berkman and Syme, 1979), the Panel Study of Income Dynamics (McDonough et al., 1997), the National Long Term Care Survey (Corder et al., 1993), the Whitehall II Study of the British Civil Service (Marmot et al., 1991), and the Malaysian Life History Survey (DaVanzo, 1984; Haaga et al., 1994).

Shifting to an emphasis on direct physiological assessment, the Framingham Study of heart disease (Allaire et al., 1999; Dawber, 1980) is an invaluable longitudinal data source with biennial physical health assessments running over 45 years. Regrettably, this rich study of physical health is nearly devoid of parallel psychosocial assessments. The implication for NIH funding priorities is that there is need to develop and maintain longitudinal studies of new birth cohorts that contain the necessary psychosocial and physiological assessments in parallel. Equally important is the need to augment judiciously selected extant surveys in the United States and other countries as the central sources for investigating inequalities in health, including assessment of predisease pathways, collective community influences, macro-level socioeconomic change, and intervening psychosocial and behavioral factors (positive and negative).

RACIAL AND ETHNIC INEQUALITY AND DISCRIMINATION

In the United States race is strongly associated with socioeconomic inequality. For example, blacks, Hispanics, and Native Americans have lower levels of income and education and higher rates of poverty and unemployment than whites. Given the strong association between race/ethnicity and SES, race/ethnicity not surprisingly is a strong predictor of health status in the United States. Moreover, available data suggest that the gap in health status between the advantaged white population and disadvantaged racial/ethnic minorities is widening over time for multiple indicators of health status (Williams, in press).

Racial/Ethnic Differences in Health Status

The association between race and health is complex and varies by the health status indicator and the particular racial group under consideration (Williams, in press). There is no generic minority health model, but all of the economically disadvantaged racial/ethnic minority populations have higher morbidity and mortality than whites for some health conditions. National mortality rates in the United States reveal that blacks consistently have higher death rates than whites for almost all the leading causes of death (National Center for Health Statistics, 1998). The notable exception to this pattern is markedly lower suicide rates for blacks compared to whites, despite rising rates of suicide over time. Hispanics consistently have lower death rates than non-Hispanic whites for the two leading causes of death in the United States (coronary heart disease and cancer) but higher death rates for several other causes of death, including diabetes, homicide, cirrhosis of the liver, and HIV/AIDS. Death rates of Hispanics exceed those of whites in the 15-44 age group (Fingerhut and Makuc, 1992). Hispanics also have elevated rates of infectious diseases such as measles, rubella, tetanus, tuberculosis, and syphilis (Vega and Amaro, 1994). Native Americans have lower death rates than whites for heart disease and cancer but higher mortality rates from injuries, flu and pneumonia, diabetes, suicide, and cirrhosis of the liver. In addition, the health status of the 60 percent of Native Americans who are covered by the Indian Health Service (a federal agency that provides medical care to Native Americans who live on or near reservations) is considerably worse than that of the national average for Native Americans (U.S. Department of Health and Human Services, 1997).

There is considerable ethnic heterogeneity within the major racial/ethnic categories. These ethnic differences predict variations in socioeconomic and demographic characteristics and access to and utilization of health care. For example, the Hispanic category encompasses more than 25 national origin groups that share a common language, religion, and traditions but that vary dramatically in terms of the timing of immigration, regional concentration, incorporation experiences, and socioeconomic status. Not surprisingly, there is considerable variation in health status within the Hispanic group (Sorlie et al., 1993; Vega and Amaro, 1994). Similarly, the Asian and Pacific Islander (API) category aggregates diverse groups from 28 Asian countries and 25 Pacific Island cultures (Lin-Fu, 1993). Although the API population has higher median income than whites, some subgroups of this population (e.g., Hmong, Laotians, and Cambodians) have poverty rates that exceed those of the black and Hispanic populations (U.S. Bureau of the Census, 1990). Although the API population has mortality rates that are markedly lower than whites, some subgroups have high rates of disease and death. For example, Native Hawaiians have the highest death rates from heart disease of any racial group in the United States (Chen, 1993) and death rates from liver cancer for Chinese Americans are four times higher than those for the white population (Lin-Fu, 1993).

Sources of Racial/Ethnic Differences in Health

Given the strong association between race/ethnicity and SES, adjusting racial disparities in health for SES sometimes eliminates but always substantially reduces these differences (Williams and Collins, 1995; Lillie-Blanton et al., 1996). However, even when education and income are held constant, blacks frequently exhibit higher levels of ill health than whites (Williams, 1996). Some studies show increasing racial differences with rising socioeconomic status (Schoendorf et al., 1992; Singh and Yu, 1995). Thus, race is more than just SES, and a growing body of research is attending to other factors associated with race that might affect health.

Racial and ethnic hierarchies usually are not clearly defined within most countries or within smaller jurisdictions, such as provinces, states, or districts. Races are socially meaningful groupings with differential access to societal resources and rewards. The basis for such hierarchies, such as they are, is usually attributed to discrimination and stigmatization of one form or another. Historically, ideologies and attitudes about racial groups translated into policies and social arrangements that limited the opportunities and life chances of stigmatized groups. The disproportionate representation of minority groups at the low end of the socioeconomic spectrum in the United States reflects social policies that limited benefits to socially marginalized groups.

The conditions of chronic discrimination in South Africa under apartheid provide an exceptionally clear picture of these relationships. In that setting, discrimination was legislated and the ordering of groups labeled "White," "Asian/Indian," "Colored," and "African"—in increasing order of formally defined discrimination—showed a clear association with mortality and a diverse set of disease categories (Singer and Ryff, 1997). Tuberculosis and TB-specific mortality were related to racial/ethnic category at both the individual and community levels throughout the apartheid period (Packard, 1989). A similar relationship is evident for HIV/AIDS from the 1980s to the present (Hope, 1999; Webb, 1997).

Racism can affect racial disparities in multiple ways. First, racial differences in socioeconomic status, one of the strongest predictors of variations in health, partly reflect the impact of economic discrimination produced by large-scale societal structures. Racial segregation determines access to educational and employment opportunities and importantly constrains socioeconomic mobility of blacks and Native Americans (Jaynes and Williams, 1987; Massey and Denton, 1993). There are racial differences in the quality of education, income returns for a given level of education or occupational status, wealth or assets associated with a given level of income, purchasing power of income, stability of employment, and health risks associated with occupational status (Williams and Collins, 1995; Kaufman et al., 1997). Health of racial/ethnic minorities can also be influenced by large-scale policy change (e.g., welfare reform), effects that warrant further scientific inquiry.

Second, segregation can affect health by creating differential neighborhood and community conditions (see Chapter 6). These include unequal access to municipal services and medical care, lower levels of social participation, higher levels of undesirable land uses, higher rates of crime, and poor-quality housing (Alba and Logan, 1993; Roberts, 1997; Shihadeh and Flynn, 1996; LeClere et al., 1997; Greenberg and Schneider, 1994). Even after adjusting for job experience and training, blacks are more likely than whites to be exposed to occupational hazards and carcinogens at work (Robinson, 1984). Hazardous waste sites are more likely to be located in poor, minority urban and rural communities than in other residential areas (Bullard, 1997; Camacho, 1998; Cole and Foster, 2000; Commission for Racial Justice, 1987).

National data reveal that blacks and Hispanics are disadvantaged compared to whites on indicators of both access to ambulatory medical care and the quality of the care received (Blendon et al., 1989; Council on Ethical and Judicial Affairs, 1990; Anderson et al., 1986; Trevino et al., 1991). Even after adjustment for health insurance and clinical status, whites are more likely than blacks to receive coronary angiography, bypass surgery, angioplasty, hemodialysis, total knee arthroplasty for osteoarthritis, intensive care for pneumonia, and kidney transplants (Giles et al., 1995; Council on Ethical and Judicial Affairs, 1990; Wilson et al., 1994).

Subjective Experience of Racism and Stigmatization

A small but growing literature indicates that chronic and acute experiences of discrimination in the lives of minority group members is a source of stress adversely affecting their physical and mental health. Laboratory studies reveal that exposure to discrimination leads to cardiovascular and psychological reactivity (Anderson, 1989; Armstead et al., 1989; Dion, 1975; Pak et al., 1991). Negative emotional responses associated with racism, particularly those that are chronic, are also associated with adverse health outcomes (Ryff and Singer, in press). Epidemiological data indicate that at least under some conditions racial discrimination is positively related to blood pressure among African Americans (Krieger, 1990; Krieger and Sidney, 1996). Other recent epidemiological studies reveal that perceptions of discrimination are adversely related to other measures of physical and mental health for a broad range of population groups (Kessler et al., 1999; Noh et al., 1999; Williams et al., 1999; Dion et al., 1992). Two recent studies have found that perceptions of discrimination make an incremental contribution over education and income in accounting for racial differences in self-reported measures of physical health (Williams et al., 1997; Ren et al., 1999).

A stigma of inferiority may create certain expectations, anxieties, and reactions that can affect the motivation, performance, and psychological well-being of some proportion of minority group members (Steele, 1997). Research across a broad range of societies reveals that socially stigmatized groups score lower on standardized tests (Fischer et al., 1996). A minority group member's endorsement of the dominant society's negative stereotype of the minority group may also have health consequences. African Americans who believe that blacks are inferior have higher levels of psychological distress and alcohol use (Taylor and Jackson, 1990; Taylor et al., 1991). The National Study of Black Americans shows that African Americans who endorse negative stereotypes of blacks as accurate are more likely to report poorer physical and mental health than those who rejected those stereotypes (Williams and Chung, in press).

Inclusion of Discrimination and Stigmatization in Longitudinal Health Studies

The National Survey of Black Americans (Jackson, 1991) provides a useful source of measures of alienation that can be linked to self-reported chronic conditions and disease. Longitudinal data are available for a subsample of this survey, and they provide a basis for constructing pathways to various health outcomes associated with perceived discrimination. The longitudinal assessments in this survey do not compare with those in the British birth cohorts or in WLS. Thus, there is a need to include a range of racial/ethnic groups in a wider array of longitudinal data bases to improve understanding of the nature and roots of health inequality.

Comparative analyses of the fine-grained assessments of perceived discrimination in African, Hispanic, and Asian subpopulations and its connection to other forms of adverse and compensating psychosocial experience have not been conducted. Although discrimination and stigmatization are associated with a range of negative health outcomes, these features have not been integrated into characterizations of the pathways of adversity and advantage across multiple life domains that lead to specification of how health outcomes come about. Understanding pathways of resilience in the face of discriminatory challenges will likely contribute important insights into why some do well and others do poorly in the face of persistent challenges.

Migration

In the United States race/ethnicity is also a strong predictor of foreign birth. A large proportion of the Hispanic and especially the Asian American populations is foreign born. The health profile of these groups reflects in part the impact of immigration. Immigrants of all racial/ethnic groups experience better health status than their native-born peers, even when these immigrants are lower in SES (Singh and Yu, 1996; Hummer et al., 1999). However, with increasing length of stay in the United States and adaptation to mainstream behavior, the health status of immigrants declines (Vega and Amaro, 1994; Marmot and Syme, 1976). For example, several behaviors that adversely affect health, such as the use of cigarettes and alcohol, have been shown to increase with length of stay and acculturation for Hispanic populations. Thus, it is likely that the health advantages evident for some subgroups of the Asian and Hispanic populations may diminish over time.

Resources

The lower levels of suicide for African Americans compared to whites is consistent with other mental health data and reflect a well-documented paradox. Blacks tend to have higher levels of ill health for most measures of physical health and are disadvantaged compared to whites on measures of subjective well-being, such as life satisfaction (Hughes and Thomas,

1998). At the same time, blacks have comparable or lower rates of psychiatric illness (Kessler et al., 1994; Robins and Regier, 1991). Thus, despite disproportionate exposure to a broad range of conditions that are risk factors for mental health problems, blacks do not have higher rates of suicide or higher rates of mental illness than whites. Similarly, although Mexican Americans are low in SES and have the lowest rates of prenatal care use of any racial/ethnic group in the United States, they have infant health outcomes that are comparable or better than that of the white population. These findings emphasize the need for research to identify the cultural strengths and health-enhancing resources resident in racial/ethnic groups. Strong family ties, religious involvement, and participation in other as yet unspecified cultural resources have been nominated as potential factors that buffer minority populations from at least some of the adverse consequences of social adversity (Williams, 1997). Research that conceptualizes and operationalizes the specific beliefs and behaviors that may be promotive of health is an important frontier of research on social inequalities and health.

RECOMMENDATIONS

Moving beyond the current NIH initiatives on socioeconomic status and health, the committee recommends the following:

- characterization of behavioral and environmental risks associated with educational, economic, and occupational disparities;
- elaboration of the subjective experiences of racism, discrimination, and stigmatization and their effects on behavior as well as their neurobiological substrates;
- assessment of health-related impacts of large-scale societal structures (e.g., racial segregation, economic discrimination, differential access to services and medical care);
- development of integrative longitudinal studies that connect the SES and racial/ethnic-related risk factors to intervening biological systems and subsequent health outcomes;
- identification of cultural strengths and health-enhancing resources resident in racial/ethnic groups and their role in accounting for resilience vis-à-vis socioeconomic inequality.

REFERENCES

Adler NE, Boyce T, Chesney MA, Cohen S, Folkman S, Kahn RL, Syme SL. 1994 "Socioeconomic status and health. The challenge of the gradient" *American Psychologist* 49/1:15-24.

Adler NE, Marmot M, McEwen BS, Stewart J (eds.). 1999 "Socioeconomic status and health in industrialized nations: Social, psychological and biological pathways" *Annals of the New York Academy of Sciences* 896.

Alba RD, Logan JR. 1993 "Minority proximity to whites in suburbs: An individual-level analysis of segregation" *American Journal of Sociology* 98/6:1388-1427.

Allaire SH, LaValley MP, Evans SR, O'Connor GT, Kelly-Hayes M, Meenan MD, Levy D, Felson DT. 1999 "Evidence for decline in disability and improved health among persons aged 55 to 70 years: The Framingham Heart Study" *American Journal of Public Health* 89/11:1678-1683.

Anderson NB. 1989 "Racial differences in stress-induced cardiovascular reactivity and hypertension: Current status and substantive issues" *Psychological Bulletin* 105/1:89-105.

Anderson RM, Giachello AL, Aday LA. 1986 "Access of Hispanics to health care and cuts in services: A state-of-the-art overview" *Public Health Reports* 101:238-252.

Antonovsky A. 1967 "Social class, life expectancy and overall mortality" *Milbank Memorial Fund Quarterly* 45:31-73.

Armstead CA, Lawler KA, Gordon G, Cross J, Gibbons J. 1989 "Relationship of racial stressors to blood pressure responses and anger expression in black college students" *Health Psychology* 8/5:541-556.

Barker DJ, Osmond C, Golding J, Kuh D, Wadsworth ME. 1989 "Growth in utero, blood pressure in childhood and adult life, and mortality from cardiovascular disease" *British Medical Association Journal* 298/6673:564-567.

Behm H. 1980. "Socioeconomic determinants of mortality in Latin America" *Population Bulletin of the United Nations* 13:1-15.

Berkman LF, Syme SL. 1979 "Social networks, host resistance, and mortality: A nine-year follow-up study of Alameda County residents" *American Journal of Epidemiology* 109/2:186-204.

Blendon RJ, Aiken LH, Freeman HE, Corey CR. 1989 "Access to medical care for black and white Americans: A matter of continuing concern" *Journal of the American Medical Association* 261/2:278-281.

Bullard RD (ed.). 1997 *Environmental Justice and Communities of Color* (San Francisco: Sierra Club Books).

Bunker JP, Gomby DS, Kehrer BH (eds.). 1989 *Pathways to Health: The Role of Social Factors* (Menlo Park CA: Henry J. Kaiser Family Foundation).

Caldji C, Tannenbaum B, Sharma S, Francis D, Plotsky PM, Meaney MJ. 1998 "Maternal care during infancy regulates the development of neural systems mediating the expression of fearfulness in the rat" *Proceedings of the National Academy of Sciences of the United States of America* 95/9:5335-5340.

Camacho D (ed.). 1998 *Environmental Injustices, Political Struggles: Race, Class and the Environment* (Durham NC: Duke University Press).

Chen MS. 1993 "A 1993 status report on the health status of Asian Pacific Islander Americans: Comparisons with Healthy People 2000 Objectives" *Asian American Pacific Islander Journal of Health* 1:37-55.

Cole L, Foster S. 2000 *From the Ground Up: Environmental Racism and the Rise of the Environmental Justice Movement* (New York: New York University Press).

Commission for Racial Justice. 1987 *Toxic Wastes and Race in the United States: A National Report on the Racial and Socio-economic Characteristics of Communities with Hazardous Waste Sites* (New York: United Church of Christ).

Corder LS, Woodbury M, Manton KG. 1993 "Health loss due to unobserved morbidity: A design based approach to minimize nonsampling error in active life expectation estimates" in JM Robine, CD Mathers, MR Bone, IR Colloque (eds.). *Calculation of Health Expectancies: Harmonization, Consensus Achieved and Future Perspectives* (Paris: INSERM) 217-232.

Council on Ethical and Judicial Affairs. 1990 "Black-white disparities in health care" *Journal of the American Medical Association* 263:2344-2346.

Danziger S, Gottschalk P (eds.). 1993 *Uneven Tides: Rising Inequality in America* (New York: Russell Sage Foundation).

DaVanzo J. 1984 "A household survey of child mortality determinants in Malaysia" *Population and Development Review* 10/suppl.:307-322.

Dawber, T. 1980 *The Framingham Study* (New York: Oxford University Press).

Deaton A. 1999 *Inequalities in Income and Inequalities in Health: NBER Working Paper 7141* (Cambridge MA: National Bureau of Economic Research).

Department of Health and Social Security. 1980 *Inequalities in Health: Report of a Research Working Group (The Black Report)* (London: Department of Health and Social Security).

Dion KL. 1975 "Women's reactions to discrimination from members of the same or opposite sex" *Journal of Research in Personality* 9/4:294-306.

Dion KL, Dion KK, Pak AW. 1992 "Personality-based hardiness as a buffer for discrimination-related stress in members of Toronto's Chinese community" *Canadian Journal of Behavioural Science* 24/4:517-536.

Duleep HO. 1989 "Measuring socioeconomic mortality differentials over time" *Demography* 26/2:345-351.

Elo IT, Preston SH. 1992 "Effects of early-life conditions on adult mortality: A review" *Population Index* 58:186-212.

Feldman JJ, Makuc DM, Kleinman JC, Cornoni-Huntley J. 1989 "National trends in educational differentials in mortality" *American Journal of Epidemiology* 129/5:919-933.

Felitti VJ, Anda RF, Nordenberg D, Williamson DF, Spitz AM, Edwards V, Koss MP, Marks JS. 1998 "Relationship of childhood abuse and household dysfunction to many of the leading causes of death in adults. The Adverse Childhood Experience (ACE) Study" *American Journal of Preventive Medicine* 14/4:245-258.

Fingerhut LA, MaKuc DM. 1992 "Mortality among minority populations in the United States" *American Journal of Public Health* 82/8:1168-1170.

Fischer CS, Hout M, Jankowski MS, Lucas SR, Swidler A, Voss K. 1996 *Inequality by Design: Cracking the Bell Curve Myth* (Princeton NJ: Princeton University Press).

Francis D, Diorio J, Liu D, Meaney MJ. 1999 "Nongenomic transmission across generations of maternal behavior and stress responses in the rat" *Science* 286/5442:1155-1158.

Garmezy N. 1993a "Children in poverty: Resilience despite risk" *Psychiatry* 56:127-136.

Garmezy N. 1993b "Vulnerability and resilience" in Funder DC, Parke RD, Tomlinson-Keasey C, Widamen K (eds.). *Studying Lives Through Time: Personality and Development* (Washington DC: American Psychological Association) 377-399.

Giles WH, Anda RF, Casper ML, Escobedo LG, Taylor HA. 1995 "Race and sex differences in rates of invasive cardiac procedures in US hospitals: Data from the National Hospital Discharge Survey" *Archives of Internal Medicine* 155/3:318-324.

Greenberg M, Schneider D. 1994 "Violence in American cities: Young black males is the answer, but what was the question?" *Social Science and Medicine* 39/2:179-187.

Grosse RN, Auffrey C. 1989 "Literacy and health status in developing countries" *Annual Review of Public Health* 10:281-297.

Haaga J, DaVanzo J, Peterson C, Peng TN. 1994 "Twelve-year follow-up of respondents in a sample survey in peninsular Malaysia" *Asia-Pacific Population Journal* 9/2:61-72.

Hauser RM, Carr D, Hauser TS, Hayes J, Krecker M, Kuo HD, Magee W, Presti J, Shinberg D, Sweeney M, Thompson-Colon TT, Uhrig N, Warren JR. 1993 "The Class of 1957 after 35 years: Overview and preliminary findings" Center for Demography and Ecology Working Paper No. 93-17, University of Wisconsin-Madison.

Hope KR (ed.). 1999 *AIDS and Development in Africa: A Social Science Perspective* (Binghamton NY: Haworth Press).

Holzer CE, Shea BM, Swanson JW, Leaf PJ, Myers J, George L, Weissman M, Bednarski P. 1986 "The increased risk for specific psychiatric disorders among persons of low socio-economic status" *American Journal of Social Psychiatry* 6/4:259-271.

Hughes M, Thomas ME. 1998 "The continuing significance of race revisited: A study of race, class, and quality of life in America, 1972 to 1996" *American Sociological Review* 63/6:785-795.

Hummer RA, Rogers RG, Nam CB, LeClere FB. 1999 "Race/ethnicity, nativity, and U.S. adult mortality" *Social Science Quarterly* 80/1:136-153.

Jackson JS. 1991 *Life in Black America* (Newbury Park CA: Sage Publications, Inc.).

Jaynes GD, Williams RM Jr. (eds.). 1987 *A Common Destiny: Blacks and American Society* (Washington DC: National Academy Press).

Kaplan GA, Pamuk ER, Lynch JW, Cohen RD, Balfour JL. 1996 "Inequality in income and mortality in the United States: Analysis of mortality and potential pathways" *British Medical Association Journal* 312/7037:999-1003.

Kaufman JS, Cooper RS, McGee DL. 1997 "Socioeconomic status and health in blacks and whites: The problem of residual confounding and the resiliency of race" *Epidemiology* 8/6:621-628.

Kessler RC, McGonagle KA, Zhao S, Nelson CB, Hughes M, Eshleman S, Wittchen H-U, Kendler KS. 1994 "Lifetime and 12-month prevalence of DSM-III-R psychiatric disorders in the United States: Results from the National Comorbidity Survey" *Archives of General Psychiatry* 51/1:8-19.

Kessler RC, Mickelson KD, Williams DR. 1999 "The prevalence, distribution, and mental health correlates of perceived discrimination in the United States" *Journal of Health and Social Behavior* 40/3:208-230.

Kitagawa EM, Hauser PM. 1973 *Differential Mortality in the United States: A Study in Socioeconomic Epidemiology* (Cambridge MA: Harvard University Press).

Korenman S, Miller JE. 1997 "Effects of long-term poverty on physical health of children in the National Longitudinal Survey of Youth" in Duncan GJ, Brooks-Gunn J (eds.). *Consequences of Growing Up Poor* (New York: Russell Sage Foundation) 70-99.

Krieger N. 1990 "Racial and gender discrimination: Risk factors for high blood pressure?" *Social Science and Medicine* 30/12:1273-1281.

Krieger N, Sidney S. 1996 "Racial discrimination and blood pressure: The CARDIA Study of young black and white adults" *American Journal of Public Health* 86/10:1370-1378.

Kunst AE, Mackenbach JP. 1994 "International variation in the size of mortality differences associated with occupational status" *International Journal of Epidemiology* 23/4:742-750.

LeClere FB, Rogers RG, Peters KD. 1997 "Ethnicity and mortality in the United States: Individual and community correlates" *Social Forces* 76/1:169-198.

Lillie-Blanton M, Parsons PE, Gayle H, Dievler A. 1996 "Racial differences in health: Not just black and white, but shades of gray" *Annual Review of Public Health* 17:411-448.

Lin-Fu JS. 1993 "Asian and Pacific Islander Americans: An overview of demographic characteristics and health care issues" *Asian and Pacific Islander Journal of Health* 1:20-36.

Liu D, Diorio J, Tannenbaum B, Caldji C, Francis D, Freedman A, Sharma S, Pearson D, Plotsky PM, Meaney MJ. 1997 "Maternal care, hippocampal glucocorticoid receptors, and hypothalamic-pituitary-adrenal responses to stress" *Science* 277/5332:1659-1662.

Lynch JW, Kaplan GA, Salonen JT. 1997a "Why do poor people behave poorly? Variation in adult health behaviours and psychosocial characteristics by stages of the socioeconomic lifecourse" *Social Science and Medicine* 44/6:809-819.

Lynch JW, Kaplan GA, Shema SJ. 1997b "Cumulative impact of sustained economic hardship on physical, cognitive, psychological, and social functioning" *New England Journal of Medicine* 337/26:1889-1895.

Lynch JW, Kaplan GA, Pamuk ER, Cohen RD, Heck KE, Balfour JL, Yen IH. 1998 "Income inequality and mortality in metropolitan areas of the United States" *American Journal of Public Health* 88/7:1074-1080.

Mackenbach JP, Stronks K, Kunst AE. 1989 "The contribution of medical care to inequalities in health: Differences between socio-economic groups in decline of mortality from conditions amenable to medical intervention" *Social Science and Medicine* 29/3:369-376.

Marmot MG, Syme SL. 1976 "Acculturation and coronary heart disease in Japanese-Americans" *American Journal of Epidemiology* 104/3:225-247.

Marmot MG, Smith GD, Stansfeld S, Patel C, North F, Head J, White I, Brunner E, Feeney A. 1991 "Health inequalities among British civil servants: The Whitehall II Study" *Lancet* 337/8754:1387-1393.

Markovic N, Bunker CH, Ukoli FA, Kuller LH. 1998 "John Henryism and blood pressure among Nigerian civil servants" *Journal of Epidemiology and Community Health* 52/3:186-90.

Massey DS, Denton NA. 1993 *American Apartheid: Segregation and the Making of the Underclass* (Cambridge MA: Harvard University Press).

McDonough P, Duncan GJ, Williams D, House J. 1997 "Income dynamics and adult mortality in the United States, 1972 through 1989" *American Journal of Public Health* 87/9:1476-1483.

McEwen BS. 1998 "Protective and damaging effects of stress mediators" *New England Journal of Medicine* 338/3:171-179.

McEwen BS, Stellar E. 1993 "Stress and the individual: Mechanisms leading to disease" *Archives of Internal Medicine* 153/18:2093-2101.

Morgenstern H. 1980 "The changing association between social status and coronary heart disease in a rural population" *Social Science and Medicine* 14A/3:191-201.

National Center for Health Statistics. 1998 *Health, United States, 1998 with Socioeconomic Status and Health Chartbook* (Hyattsville MD: U.S. Department of Health and Human Services).

Noh S, Beiser M, Kaspar V, Hou F, Rummens J. 1999 "Perceived racial discrimination, depression, and coping: A study of Southeast Asian refugees in Canada" *Journal of Health and Social Behavior* 40/3:193-207.

Packard RM. 1989 *White Plague, Black Labor: Tuberculosis and the Political Economy of Health and Disease in South Africa* (Berkeley: University of California Press).

Pak AW, Dion KL, Dion KK. 1991 "Social-psychological correlates of experienced discrimination: Test of the double jeopardy hypothesis" *International Journal of Intercultural Relations* 15/2:243-254.

Pappas G, Queen S, Hadden W, Fisher G. 1993 "The increasing disparity in mortality between socioeconomic groups in the United States, 1960 and 1986" *New England Journal of Medicine* 329/2:103-109.

Power C, Matthews S. 1997 "Origins of health inequalities in a national population sample" *Lancet* 350/9091:1584-1589.

Ren XS, Amick BC, Williams DR. 1999 "Racial/ethnic disparities in health: The interplay between discrimination and socioeconomic status" *Ethnicity and Disease* 9/2:151-165.

Roberts EM. 1997 "Neighborhood social environments and the distribution of low birthweight in Chicago" *American Journal of Public Health* 87/4:597-603.

Robins LN, Regier DA (eds.). 1991 *Psychiatric Disorders in America: The Epidemiologic Catchment Area Study* (New York: Free Press).

Robinson J. 1984 "Racial inequality and the probability of occupation-related injury or illness" *Milbank Memorial Fund Quarterly* 62:567-593.

Ryff CD, Singer B. 2000 "Interpersonal flourishing: A positive health agenda for the new millennium" *Personality and Social Psychology Review* 4:30-44.

Ryff CD, Singer B. In press "The role of emotion on pathways to positive health" in RJ Davidson, HH Goldsmith, K. Scherer (eds.). *Handbook of Affective Science* (New York: Oxford University Press).

Ryff CD, Singer B, Love GD, Essex MJ. 1998 "Resilience in adulthood and later life: Defining features and dynamic processes" in Lomranz J (ed.). *Handbook of Aging and Mental Health: An Integrative Approach* (New York: Plenum Press) 69-96.

Schoendorf KC, Hogue CJ, Kleinman JC, Rowley D. 1992 "Mortality among infants of black as compared with white college-educated parents" *New England Journal of Medicine* 326/23:1522-1526.

Seeman TE, Singer BH, Rowe JW, Horwitz RI, McEwen BS. 1997 "Price of adaptation—allostatic load and its health consequences: MacArthur studies of successful aging" *Archives of Internal Medicine* 157/19:2259-2268.

Shihadeh ES, Flynn N. 1996 "Segregation and crime: The effect of black social isolation on the rates of black urban violence" *Social Forces* 74/4:1325-1352.

Singer B, Ryff CD. 1997 "Racial and ethnic inequalities in health: Environmental, psychosocial, and physiological pathways" in Devlin B, Fienberg SE, Resnick DP, Roeder K (eds.). *Intelligence, Genes, and Success: Scientists Respond to the Bell Curve* (New York: Springer) 89-122.

Singer B, Ryff CD. 1999. "Hierarchies of life histories and associated health risks" *Annals of the New York Academy of Sciences* 896:96-115.

Singer B, Ryff CD, Carr D, Magee WJ. 1998 "Linking life histories and mental health: A person-centered strategy" in Raftery A (ed.). *Sociological Methodology* (Washington DC: American Sociological Association) 1-51.

Singh GK, Yu SM. 1995 "Infant mortality in the United States: Trends, differentials, and projections, 1950 through 2010" *American Journal of Public Health* 85/7:957-964.

Singh GK, Yu SM. 1996. "Adverse pregnancy outcomes: Differences between US- and foreign-born women in major US racial and ethnic groups" *American Journal of Public Health* 86/6:837-843.

Smith, JP. 1999 "Healthy bodies and thick wallets: The dual relation between health and economic status." *Journal of Economic Perspectives* 13/2:145-166.

Sorlie PD, Backlund E, Johnson NJ, Rogot E. 1993 "Mortality by Hispanic status in the United States" *Journal of the American Medical Association* 270/20:2464-2468.

Sorokin, PA. 1927 *Social Mobility* (New York: Harper & Brothers).

Steele CM. 1997 "A threat in the air: How stereotypes shape intellectual identity and performance" *American Psychologist* 52/6:613-629.

Taylor J, Jackson B. 1990 "Factors affecting alcohol consumption in black women: Part II" *International Journal of the Addictions* 25/12:1415-1427.

Taylor J, Henderson D, Jackson BB. 1991 "A holistic model for understanding and predicting depressive symptoms in African-American women" *Journal of Community Psychology* 19/4:306-320.

Trevino FM, Moyer ME, Valdez RB, Stroup-Benham CA. 1991 "Health insurance coverage and utilization of health services by Mexican Americans, mainland Puerto Ricans, and Cuban Americans" *Journal of the American Medical Association* 265/2:233-237.

U.S. Bureau of the Census. 1990 *Census of Population and Housing, 1990: County Population by Age, Sex, Race, and Spanish Origin* (Washington DC: Data User Services).

U.S. Department of Health and Human Services, Indian Health Service. 1997 *Regional Differences in Indian Health* (Rockville MD: U.S. Department of Health and Human Services).

Vega WA, Amaro H. 1994 "Latino outlook: Good health, uncertain prognosis" *Annual Review of Public Health* 15:39-67.

Wadsworth ME, Kuh DJ. 1997 "Childhood influences on adult health: A review of recent work from the British 1946 national birth cohort study, the MRC National Survey of Health and Development" *Pediatric and Perinatal Epidemiology* 11/1:2-20.

Webb D. 1997 *HIV and AIDS in Africa* (London: Pluto Press).

Wilkinson RG. 1986 *Class and Health: Research and Longitudinal Data* (London: Tavistock Publications).

Wilkinson RG. 1994. *Unfair Shares: The Effects of Widening Income Differences on the Welfare of the Young* (Ilford, U.K.:   Bernardo's).

Williams DR. 1990 "Socioeconomic differentials in health: A review and redirection" *Social Psychology Quarterly* 53/2:81-99.

Williams DR. 1996 "Race/ethnicity and socioeconomic status: Measurement and methodological issues" *International Journal of Health Services* 26/3:483-505.

Williams DR. 1997 "Race and health: Basic questions, emerging directions" *Annals of Epidemiology* 7/5:322-333.

Williams DR. 2001 "Racial variations in adult health status: Patterns, paradoxes and prospects" in Smelser N, Wilson WJ, Mitchell F (eds.). *America Becoming: Racial Trends and Their Consequences* (Washington DC: National Academy Press):371-410.

Williams DR, Chung A-M. In press "Racism and health" in Gibson R, Jackson JS (eds.). *Health in Black America* (Thousand Oaks CA: Sage Publications).

Williams DR, Collins C. 1995 "U.S. socioeconomic and racial differences in health: Patterns and explanations" *Annual Review of Sociology* 21:349-386.

Williams DR, Yu Y, Jackson J, Anderson N. 1997 "Racial differences in physical and mental health: Socioeconomic status, stress, and discrimination" *Journal of Health Psychology* 2/3:335-51.

Williams DR, Spencer MS, Jackson JS. 1999 "Race, stress, and physical health: The role of group identity" in Contrada RJ, Ashmore RD (eds.). *Self, Social Identity, and Physical Health: Interdisciplinary Explorations* (New York: Oxford University Press) 71-100.

Wilson MG, May DS, Kelly JJ. 1994 "Racial differences in the use of total knee arthroplasty for osteoarthritis among older Americans" *Ethnicity and Disease* 4/1:57-67.

8
Population Perspectives: Understanding Health Trends and Evaluating the Health Care System

The earlier chapters on predisease pathways, positive health, environmentally induced gene expression, and personal ties place strong emphasis on preventing disease, maintaining allostasis, and promoting well-being at levels comparatively proximal to the individual (social, psychological, neurophysiological). The chapters addressing collective properties of communities and inequality focus on more intermediate levels whereby environmental and social structural factors influence health. This chapter focuses explicitly on questions of population health at the macro level. Four primary issues are considered: (1) time trends and spatial variation in population health; (2) accounting for such trends, with particular emphasis given to social and behavioral factors; (3) understanding links between population health and the macroeconomy; and (4) evaluating the health care system. An important crosscutting research priority, among several others delineated below, is to account for population health processes by linking them via multilevel analyses to behavioral, psychosocial, and environmental factors described in earlier chapters.

TIME TRENDS AND SPATIAL VARIATION IN POPULATION HEALTH

Brief summaries are provided below of health trends in life expectancy and disability, both within the United States and in other countries. Changing rates of communicable diseases (e.g., sexually transmitted diseases and tuberculosis) are also examined. Finally, various indicators of child health (e.g., infant mortality, birth weight, asthma, and other respiratory conditions) are reviewed. Some of these population trends show health improvements across time; others point to increasing health problems. Behavioral and psychosocial factors are implicated in both. A major international data source on health trends is the set of Demographic and Health Surveys.[1] An overarching theme is that the maintenance and improvement of population health have been and continue to be due as much to changes in broader socioeconomic and environmental forces as to more microscopically based biobehavioral science. Understanding and facilitating improvements in socioeconomic conditions, general public health and sanitation, and private and public policies affecting lifestyle have accounted for the bulk of historical changes in population health and very likely recent advances as well (Rose, 1992).

Life Expectancy

Health varies substantially across and within countries. For example, in 1998 life expectancy in Sierra Leone was 37 years and in Japan it was 80 years. Ninety percent of this range, however, is covered by variation across counties within the United States. The range in life expectancy between females born in Stearns County, Minnesota, and males born in various counties in South Dakota is 22.5 years and extends to 41.3 years when race-specific life expectancy is calculated (WHO, 1999). Over time, life expectancy in the United States has risen from 47 years in 1900 to 78 years in 1995. Table 1 shows the changes in life expectancy at birth between approximately 1910 and 1998 in selected countries.

On average, people in richer countries live longer and have higher-quality lives than people in poorer countries. Within countries, at the city, county, and regional levels, people with higher socioeconomic status are on average in better health than those with lower socioeconomic status. As described in Chapter 7, there is also considerable variation across racial and ethnic categories that interacts with socioeconomic status.

Disability

Recent research shows clearly that chronic disease disability rates are falling in the United States. Figure 1 shows the proportion of the elderly who were disabled in 1982, 1984, 1989, and 1994. Disability is measured as impairments in activities of daily living (ADLs, such as bathing, toileting)

---

[1]The data are available electronically: Demographic and Health Surveys: http://www.measuredhs.com.

TABLE 1 Life Expectancy at Birth for Selected Countries

Country	Around 1910		1998	
	Males	Females	Males	Females
Australia	56	60	75	81
Chile	29	33	72	78
England and Wales	49	53	75	80
Italy	46	47	75	81
Japan	43	43	77	83
New Zealand[a]	60	63	74	80
Norway	56	59	75	81
Sweden	57	59	76	81
United States	49	53	73	80

[a]Excluding Maoris.
SOURCE: WHO, 1999.

or instrumental activities of daily living (IADLs, such as the ability to perform light household work, use the telephone). The data, from the National Long-Term Care Survey, are for a representative sample of the elderly in each year. The questions are the same in each survey, so the responses give the most accurate available measure of changes in disability over time.

In 1982 and 1984 nearly 25 percent of the elderly were disabled. By 1994 disability had declined to 21 percent, a reduction of over 1 percent per year. Furthermore, disability decline is more rapid in the second half of the time period (1989-1994) than the first half (1984-1989). These findings have been confirmed in other data as well (Freedman and Martin, 1998), suggesting the trend is not an artifact of this particular sample.

Sketchier evidence suggests that the decline in elderly disability has occurred throughout the developed world. Rates of disability and institutionalization among the elderly in various developed countries, compiled by the Organization for Economic Cooperation and Development (Jacobzone, 2000), have been declining over time in most countries. The decline is only modest in some countries (e.g., the United Kingdom) but is rapid in others (e.g., Japan). The average rate of decline among countries where disability rates are falling is 2.3 percent per year. In only two countries have rates of severe disability increased (Australia and Canada), but even there the rates of institutionalization are falling. Such rates have been falling as well in four of the five countries for which there are time series data, although the decline is generally less rapid than the decline in the rate of severe disability. The exception is France, where institutionalization rates have been increas-

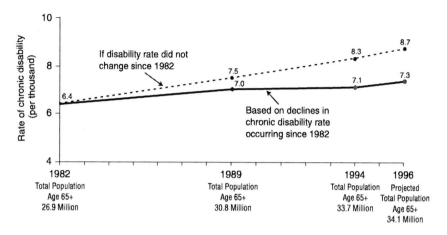

FIGURE 1 Changes in chronic disability among the elderly, 1982-1996.
SOURCE: Manton et al. (1997).

ing, perhaps reflecting a change in the location of care. Rates of severe disability in France, however, are declining rapidly.

Overall, these changes in disability have been sufficiently large for some to argue that health promotion might solve the long-term problems of financing public medical care systems (Singer and Manton, 1998). Behavioral, environmental, and psychosocial factors are, as we argue throughout this report, key routes to such health promotion.

Communicable Diseases

Sexually transmitted diseases (STDs) and tuberculosis are among the most important communicable diseases in the United States. The incidence of reported chlamydial infections and viral STDs has steadily increased in recent years, while the incidence of gonorrhea has generally declined. Levels of syphilis vary among different population subgroups but have reached record lows since 1995. Vaginal infections such as trichomonas and bacterial vaginosis have probably remained high, although surveillance for these conditions is rudimentary. Table 2 shows the estimated incidence and prevalence of STDs in the United States in 1996.[2]

The number of reported cases of gonorrhea has generally declined,

---

[2]The full report is available online from the Kaiser Family Foundation: http://www.kff.org/content/archive/1447/std_rep.pdf.

TABLE 2 Estimated Incidence and Prevalence of Sexually
Transmitted Diseases in the United States, 1996

Sexually Transmitted Diseases	Incidence	Prevalence
Chlamydia	3 million	2 million
Gonorrhea	650,000	—
Syphilis	70,000	—
Herpes	1 million	45 million
Human papilloma virus	5.5 million	20 million
Hepatitis B	77,000	750,000
Trichamoniasis	5 million	—
Bacterial vaginosis	No estimate	—
HIV	20,000	560,000

SOURCE: Kaiser Family Foundation, 1998.

starting in the mid-1970s with the introduction of the national gonorrhea control program. A disproportionate share of the decline occurred among older white populations, with infection rates remaining relatively high among minority groups and adolescents. In 1996 the Centers for Disease Control and Prevention (CDC) reported 325,000 new cases of gonorrhea (CDC, 1999b). Because previous investigations have shown that only about half of all diagnosed gonorrhea cases are reported to public health authorities, total gonorrhea infections are estimated to be 650,000 in Table 2.

HIV infection trends in the United States show that in the mid-1970s HIV was transmitted primarily among homosexual and bisexual men. The virus entered the injection-drug-using populations in the 1980s and rapidly spread during that decade. Limited heterosexual transmission occurred until the 1980s. Since 1989 the greatest proportional increase in reported AIDS cases has been among heterosexuals, with this trend expected to continue (Rosenberg, 1995). New methods of estimating HIV incidence and prevalence (Holmberg, 1996) yielded an estimate of 41,000 new HIV infections annually, with between 700,000 and 800,000 prevalent HIV infections. The introduction of protease inhibitors may increase the number of prevalent infections by extending the life of HIV-infected people. Approximately half of the incident and three-quarters of prevalent infections were estimated to have been sexually transmitted. Globally, the incidence of HIV is much higher than in the United States, with an estimated 5.8 million new infections annually and more than 30 million persons currently living with HIV (UNAIDS, 1998). More than 90 percent of the global total has been spread sexually.

An important priority for future research is to improve the accuracy of these estimates. Most STD incidence and prevalence estimates are derived from multiple populations, few of which are representative national surveys, such as NHANES or the national reporting system for AIDS. Establishing nationally representative surveillance for the full range of STDs would help narrow the uncertainty in current estimates. For example, the true number of STD infections could be as low as 10 million or as high as 20 million. The current point estimate is 15.3 million.

Potential improvement in the U.S. STD epidemic could ensue from full implementation of the national prevention and control program identified by the expert panel assembled by the Institute of Medicine (Eng and Butler, 1997). The program focuses on improving public awareness and education, reaching adolescents and women, and instituting effective culturally appropriate programs to promote healthy behavior by adolescents and adults. Additional targets are integrating public health programs, training health care professionals, and modifying messages from the mass media. Improved surveillance of STD incidence and prevalence rates will be necessary to document the progress of such initiatives.

Turning to global tuberculosis, 6.7 million new cases and 2.4 million deaths were estimated in 1998 (Murray and Salomon, 1998). Based on current tends in implementation of the World Health Organization's strategy of directly observed, short-course treatment, a total of 225 million new cases and 79 million deaths from tuberculosis are expected between 1998 and 2030 (Murray and Salomon, 1998). Active case finding using mass miniature radiography could save 23 million lives over this period, which underscores the importance of prevention. Single-contact treatments for TB could avert 24 million new cases and 11 million deaths. Combined with active screening, single-contact treatments could reduce TB mortality by 40 percent.

In the United States the situation is quite different. Table 3 shows the number of reported cases of TB from 1975 to 1992 (CDC, 1999d). The rapid decline in TB cases from 1975 to 1986 was followed by an increase through 1991. However, in 1998 a total of 18,361 TB cases were reported in the 50 states and the District of Columbia, a decrease of 8 percent from 1997 and 31 percent from 1992, the height of the TB resurgence. The 1998 rate of 6.8 per 100,000 population was 35 percent lower than in 1992 (10.5) but remained above the national goal for 2000 of 3.5 per 100,000 (CDC, 1999a).

Considering infectious diseases more generally and on a longer time scale, infectious disease mortality declined during the first eight decades of the twentieth century from 797 deaths per 100,000 people in 1900 to 36 deaths per 100,000 in 1980. The overall general decline was interrupted by a sharp increase in mortality due to the 1918 influenza epidemic. From 1938 to 1952 the decline was particularly rapid, with mortality decreasing by 8.2 percent per year. Pneumonia and influenza were responsible for the

TABLE 3 Tuberculosis Cases, Case Rates, Deaths, and Death Rates per 100,000 Population: United States, 1975-1998

Year	Tuberculosis Cases				Tuberculosis Deaths			
			Percent Change				Percent Change	
	Number	Rate^a	Number	Rate	Number	Rate^a	Number	Rate
1975	33,989	15.9	—	—	3,333	1.6	-5.1	-5.9
1976	32,105	15.0	-5.5	-5.7	3,130	1.5	-6.1	-6.3
1977	30,145	13.9	-6.1	-7.3	2,968	1.4	-5.2	-6.7
1978	28,521	13.1	-5.4	-5.8	2,914	1.3	-1.8	-7.1
1979	27,669	12.6	-3.0	-3.8	2,007^b	0.9^b	-31.^b	-30.8^b
1980	27,749	12.3	+0.3	-2.4	1,978	0.9	-1.4	0.0
1981	27,373	11.9	-1.4	-3.3	1,937	0.8	-2.1	-11.1
1982	25,520	11.0	-6.8	-7.6	1,807	0.8	-6.7	0.0
1983	23,846	10.2	-6.6	-7.3	1,779	0.8	-1.5	0.0
1984	22,255	9.4	-6.7	-7.8	1,729	0.7	-2.8	-12.5
1985	22,201	9.3	-0.2	-1.1	1,752	0.7	+1.3	0.0
1986	22,768	9.4	+2.6	+1.1	1,782	0.7	+1.7	0.0
1987	22,517	9.3	-1.1	-1.1	1,755	0.7	-1.5	0.0
1988	22,436	9.1	-0.4	-2.2	1,921	0.8	+9.5	+14.3
1989	23,495	9.5	+4.7	+4.4	1,970	0.8	+2.6	0.0
1990	25,701	10.3	+9.4	+8.4	1,810	0.7	-8.1	-12.5
1991	26,283	10.4	+2.3	+1.0	1,713	0.7	-5.4	0.0
1992	26,673	10.5	+1.5	+1.0	1,705	0.7	-0.5	0.0
1993	25,287	9.8	-5.2	'-6.7	1,631	0.6	-4.3	-14.3
1994	24,361	9.4	-3.7	-4.1	1,478	0.6	-9.4	0.0
1995	22,860	8.7	-6.2	-7.4	1,336	0.5	-9.6	-16.7
1996	21,337	8.0	-6.7	-8.0	1,202	0.5	-10.0	0.0
1997	19,851	7.4	-7.0	-7.5	1,166	0.4	-3.0	-20.0
1998	18,361	6.8	-7.5	-8.1	...	...	...	...

^aPer 100,000 population.
^bThe large decrease in 1979 occurred because late effects of tuberculosis (e.g., bronchiectasis or fibrosis) and pleurisy with effusion (without mention of cause) are no longer included in tuberculosis deaths. Ellipses indicate data are not available.
SOURCE: Data from CDC, 1999d, Table 1.

largest number of infectious disease deaths throughout the century. Although tuberculosis caused almost as many deaths as pneumonia and influenza early in the century, TB mortality dropped off sharply after 1945. Infectious disease mortality increased in the 1980s and early 1990s in persons aged 25 years and older, due mainly to the emergence of AIDS in 25- to 64-year-olds and to a lesser degree to increases in influenza and pneumonia deaths in persons aged 65 and older. Although most of the twentieth century was marked by declining infectious disease mortality, substantial year-to-year variations and recent increases emphasize the dynamic nature of infectious diseases and the need for preparedness to address them. A considerable effort in this direction was stimulated by a 1992 Institute of Medicine (IOM) report focused on emerging infectious diseases. A wider-ranging multidisciplinary program emphasizing emerging infectious diseases of wildlife, including threats to human health, (Daszak et al., 2000) is notable for its integrative consideration of ecology, pathology, and population biology of host-parasite systems and the emphasis on investigations incorporating individual, population, and environmental perspectives.

Child Health

In the United States the overall infant mortality rate has decreased rapidly since 1960. Between 1960 and 1994 the rate fell from 24.9 to 8.0 infant deaths per 1,000 live births. Between 1960 and 1992 the infant mortality rate decreased by 69 percent among whites, 62 percent among African Americans, 68 percent among Asians, and 77 percent among Native Americans. Nevertheless, as of 1992 there were considerable racial and ethnic disparities in the infant mortality rate (see also Chapter 7). The African American infant mortality rate of 16.8 infant deaths per 1,000 live births was 2.4 times higher than the white rate of 6.9. The Native American rate of 9.9 infant deaths per 1,000 live births was second highest, and the Asian rate of 4.8 per 1,000 live births was lowest.

Two other trends of concern in the health of children that are implicated in longer-term negative health consequences are the rate of low-birth-weight babies and the teen birth rate. Nationally, the percent of live births weighing less than 5.5 lbs. (a standard indicator of low birth weight) was 6.8 in 1985 and 7.4 in 1996. The number of births to teenagers between 15 and 17 per 1,000 females in this age category rose from 31 in 1985 to 34 in 1996. There was substantial variation across states in these two statistics. For example, in 1996 the low-birth-weight rate was 4.8 percent in New Hampshire, 9.9 percent in Mississippi, and 14.3 percent in the District of Columbia. The teen birth rate ranged from 15 in New Hampshire to 52 in Mississippi and 79 in the District of Columbia (Annie E. Casey Foundation, 1999).

When assessing the health of children, it is important to examine the prevalence of chronic health conditions. Children with persistent health problems are more likely to miss school and require medical assistance and follow-up. Such chronic problems also pose difficulties for the parents, who may experience emotional stress, often lose days from work, and incur additional medical expenses associated with recurrent medical visits and follow-up care. The circumstances of both children and their parents in this kind of persistent difficult environment contribute to the predisease pathways described in Chapter 2.

Asthma is the most common chronic disease of childhood, affecting an estimated 4.8 million children. It is one of the leading causes of school absenteeism, accounting for over 10 million missed school days each year (U.S. DHHS, 1996). In addition, managing asthma is expensive and imposes financial burdens on the families of people who have it. In 1990 the cost of asthma to the U.S. economy was estimated to be $6.2 billion, with the majority of the expense attributed to medical care. A 1996 analysis found the annual cost of asthma to be $14 billion (CECS, 1998).

Table 4 shows the number of children per 1,000 children aged 0-17 in 1993 with a diversity of chronic conditions (NCHS, 1993). Over the past 20 years, respiratory conditions have been the most prevalent type of chronic health problem experienced by children aged 0-17. Rates for most of the chronic health problems identified in Table 4 were fairly constant during that time period, with the exception of chronic respiratory conditions, which showed sizable increases from 1982 to 1993. For example, rates of chronic bronchitis rose from 34 per 1,000 children in 1982 to 59 per 1,000 in 1993 (a 76 percent increase). Similarly, rates of asthma rose 79 percent, going from 40 cases per 1,000 in 1982 to 72 cases per 1,000 in 1993 (NCHS, 1982-1993).

Risk Factors

In a widely cited paper McGinnis and Foege (1993) showed that unhealthy behaviors and environmental exposures were the "actual causes of death" that accounted for 50 percent of all U.S. mortality. Heading the list of causes were tobacco (19 percent), diet/activity patterns (14 percent), and alcohol (5 percent). Smoking has transformed lung cancer from a virtually unknown disease in 1900 to the leading cause of cancer deaths in 1999, accounting with environmental tobacco smoke and interactions with other exposures (e.g., radon) for more than 90 percent of lung cancer deaths each year. Smoking is also the leading cause of chronic obstructive pulmonary disease and chronic bronchitis and emphysema (Warner, 2000). The prevalence of smoking has dropped from 45 percent in 1963, the year prior to publication of the Surgeon General's report on smoking and health (U.S.

TABLE 4 Selected Reported Chronic Conditions, Number per 1,000 Persons, by Age: United States, 1993

Type of Chronic Condition	All Ages	Under 18 Years
Selected conditions of the genitourinary, nervous, endocrine, metabolic, and blood-forming systems:		
Goiter or other disorders of the thyroid	16.3	1.9
Diabetes	30.7	1.5
Anemias	15.4	8.6
Epilepsy	5.3	5.4
Migraine headache	43.3	13.2
Neuralgia or neuritis, unspecified	2.7	0.2
Kidney trouble	15.1	4.7
Bladder disorders	15.8	3.4
Diseases of the prostate	8.0	–
Disease of female genital organs	21.0	2.6
Selected circulatory conditions:		
Rheumatic fever with or without heart disease	7.9	1.2
Heart disease	83.6	20.3
Ischemic heart disease	28.1	0.3
Heart rhythm disorders	35.9	14.9
Tachycardia or rapid heart	8.7	0.4
Heart murmurs	19.5	14.1
Other and unspecified heart rhythm disorders	7.6	0.5
Other selected diseases of the heart, excluding hypertension	19.6	5.0
High blood pressure (hypertension)	108.3	3.1
Cerebrovascular disease	13.2	1.0
Hardening of the arteries	7.0	–
Varicose veins of the lower extremities	30.0	0.6
Hemorrhoids	39.8	0.2
Selected respiratory conditions:		
Chronic bronchitis	54.3	59.3
Asthma	51.4	71.6
Hay fever or allergic rhinitis without asthma	93.4	56.7
Chronic sinusitis	146.7	79.6
Deviated nasal septum	7.0	0.7
Chronic disease of the tonsils or adenoids	11.0	26.4
Emphysema	7.6	0.7

SOURCE: Data from NCHS, 1993.

DHEW, 1964), to 25 percent in 1997 (CDC, 1999c). Based on projections of the demographics of smoking, even in the absence of stronger tobacco control education and policy, and assuming no change in youth initiation of smoking, prevalence should continue to fall over the next 20 years, leveling off at approximately 18 percent of adults (Mendez and Warner, 1998; see also Chapter 9).

Of adult Americans, 24.7 percent were smokers in 1997 (CDC, 1999c). Although a greater percentage of men smoke than women (27.6 percent and 22.1 percent, respectively), the gap between the two genders has declined gradually over time. Racial and ethnic differences in smoking prevalence are substantial, ranging from 16.9 percent for Asians and Pacific Islanders to 34.1 percent for Native Americans and Native Alaskans. Smoking rates vary substantially by age, with prevalence declining in the fourth and subsequent decades of life. Smoking cessation, the principal determinant of the decline in prevalence with age, rises significantly with age.

An important research challenge for demographers is the development of more effective ways of assessing smoking initiation. In the 1999 Monitoring the Future Survey, 34.6 percent of high school seniors had smoked within the previous 30 days.[3] The comparable figures for tenth and eighth graders were 25.7 percent and 17.5 percent, respectively. The interpretive problem with these figures, from the point of view of health risk, is that, while 30-day prevalence rates were rising during the 1990s, measures of regular and heavy smoking (e.g., half a pack or more per day) were not. While the latter clearly point to increased health risk, it is unclear what risks follow from the 30-day prevalence rates among youth.

Since the inception of the antismoking campaign in 1964, the most notable change in smoking prevalence is by education class. In 1965, the year following the first Surgeon General's report, less than 3 percentage points separated the prevalence of smoking among college graduates (33.7 percent) from that of Americans who did not graduate from high school (U.S. DHHS, 1989). By 1997 prevalence among college graduates had fallen by nearly two-thirds to 11.6 percent. Among people without a high school diploma, in contrast, prevalence had fallen by only one-sixth (to 30.4 percent; CDC, 1999c; Warner, 2000). Although considerable speculation has been put forth about the reasons for this disparity, this is an important future research direction, directly linked to those of Chapter 6 and Chapter 7, where the social and behavioral sciences are particularly prominent.

Dietary factors and sedentary activity patterns together account for at least 300,000 deaths each year (McGinnis and Foege, 1993). Dietary fac-

---

[3]The data are available electronically: http://monitoringthefuture.org/.

tors have been associated with cardiovascular diseases (coronary artery disease, stroke, and hypertension), cancers (colon, breast, and prostate), and diabetes mellitus (U.S. DHHS, 1988). Physical inactivity has been associated with an increased risk for heart disease (Manson et al., 1992; Paffenberger et al., 1990) and colon cancer (Lee et al., 1991). The interdependence of dietary factors and physical activity patterns as risk factors for obesity has received considerable attention (Mokdad et al., 1999; Wickelgren, 1998; Hill and Peters, 1998; Tauber, 1998). Understanding these interactions as part of a more mechanistic characterization of pre-disease pathways (Chapter 2) to a range of cardiovascular diseases and cancers is an important research direction requiring integrative perspectives (see Chapter 1).

Alcohol and illicit drug use are associated with violence, injury (particularly automobile injuries and fatalities), and HIV infection (injecting drugs with contaminated needles). The annual economic costs to the United States from alcohol abuse are estimated to be $167 billion, and the costs from drug abuse are estimated to be $110 billion (U.S. DHHS, 2000). Among adolescents alcohol is the most frequently used substance among the alcohol/illicit drug items. In 1997, 21 percent of adolescents aged 12-17 years reported drinking alcohol in the last month. Such use has remained at about 20 percent since 1992. Eight percent of this age group reported binge drinking and 3 percent were heavy drinkers (five or more drinks on the same occasion on each of five or more days in the last 30 days). Data from 1998 show that 10 percent of adolescents aged 12-17 years reported using illicit drugs in the last 30 days. This rate is significantly lower than in the previous year and remains well below the all-time high of 16 percent in 1979. Current illicit drug use had nearly doubled for those aged 12 to 13 years between 1996 and 1997 but then decreased between 1997 and 1998. Among adults binge drinking has remained at the same approximate level of 16 percent since 1988, with the highest current rate of 32 percent among adults aged 18 to 25 years. Illicit drug use has been near the present rate of 6 percent since 1980. Men continue to have higher rates of illicit drug use than women, and rates are higher in urban than in rural areas (U.S. DHHS, 2000).

The above data summarize population-level profiles of adverse health behaviors (smoking, obesity and physical inactivity, alcohol and illicit drug use). Consistent with the integrative theme guiding this report (see Chapter 1), there is a great need for broadening research agendas around these topics. On the one hand, the behavioral and social sciences can help identify precursors (e.g., personality factors, coping styles, socialization processes, work and family stress, peer and community influences) to poor health practices (see Chapters 2, 5, and 6). Understanding the mechanisms through which poor health behaviors translate to chronic disease requires, however, that the above processes be linked to gene expression and multiple pathophysiological systems. It also requires attending to the reality that many of the above risk factors (behavioral and physiological) co-occur and have multiple health consequences (see discussion of co-occurring risk and comorbidity in Chapter 2).

From the integrative perspective, it is important to recognize that many of the above behavioral, psychological, social, and environmental factors are driven by broad social structural influences, such as socioeconomic inequality and racial/ethnic discrimination and stigmatization (see Chapter 7). Thus, macro-level forces must also be part of the integrative agenda. Finally, from the perspectives of prevention and treatment, the social and behavioral sciences point to diverse venues for avoiding, offsetting, or reversing these poor health practices (see Chapters 3 and 9). This report calls for deeper understanding of these interacting processes and thus requires coming at the question of population health risk from many diverse but related angles.

ACCOUNTING FOR MACRO-LEVEL HEALTH PATTERNS

An integrative perspective is required both to understand the antecedents and consequents of behavioral health risks and to account for macro-level changes in health, such as gains in life expectancy, declining rates of disability, the spread of STDs, and infant mortality and childhood diseases. These topics and needed agendas following from them are described below.

Life Expectancy

The dramatic increase in life expectancy in the United States during the twentieth century is attributable largely to primary prevention interventions (Bloom, 1999), such as improved sanitation, housing, nutrition, and new technologies for food preservation. The decrease of 6 percent per decade in chronic disease prevalence in males between 1910 and 1985 was achieved with relatively primitive medical and public health technologies and when little was known about the mechanisms of chronic disease processes at relatively advanced ages (Fogel, 1999). Recent data suggest that nutritional factors affecting maternal health and fetal development help explain this chronic disease risk decline (Fogel, 1999). Nutritional deficiencies could have affected maternal pelvic development and increased subsequent risks for cerebrovascular disease in the 1910 elderly Civil War veteran cohorts who were born between 1825 and 1844 (Costa, 1998). Maternal nutritional deficiency during pregnancy also can impact development of the pancreas and liver in the fetus, which may alter risks of diabetes and heart disease as the child ages. These nutritional deficiencies were increasingly alleviated in the post-1840s birth cohorts.

Chronic disease risks were further altered in the early part of the twentieth century. For example, in the 1920s and 1930s changes in food preservation, thermal preparation, and storage affecting microbial food contaminants likely combined with changes in salt intake and water quality (e.g., reducing the prevalence of *H. pylori* infections) to alter the incidence of a wide range of chronic diseases, including stroke, hypertension, gastric and other cancers, and peptic ulcers (Fogel, 1999; Fogel and Costa, 1997). A similar pattern was found in Great Britain. Up to the 1940s the British centenarian population grew 1 percent per year (Perutz, 1998). After the 1940s (i.e., centenarians born after the 1840s) the growth rate was nearer 6 percent. Thus, in both Britain and the United States the major socioeconomic and nutritional changes appear to have affected the health and survival of post-1840 birth cohorts.

The national trends described above are accompanied by enormous variation within countries. County-specific analyses of historical trends in the adoption of primary prevention strategies and shifts in average socioeconomic status levels relative to those for a given state, or for the country at large, could provide a useful baseline for the formulation and targeting of future health promotion and disease prevention strategies.

Disability

Several influences on declining rates of disability among the elderly have been proposed. One suggestion is that these health improvements result from changes in the nature of work. Work has become less manually intensive and more cognitive over time, potentially delaying the onset of a range of adverse conditions, including musculoskeletal disorders and cardiovascular complications. In addition, exposure to dust and hazardous chemicals has declined. Preliminary evidence suggests that these changes may explain up to one-quarter of improvements in health for the elderly since the turn of the century (Costa, 1998), although no evidence exists for recent years.

The nature of work may matter in other ways as well. Work that is mentally stressful or not mentally challenging enough may lead to psychological stress that is manifest in physical disorder. For example, musculoskeletal disorders are more common in people with low job satisfaction, elevated psychophysiological stress reactions, and lack of opportunity to unwind, all of which are characteristic of repetitious work with short time cycles (Melin and Lundberg, 1997). Such findings are also reported in the Whitehall studies (Marmot et al., 1991; Marmot, 1994).

A second possibility is that health improvements result from improved socioeconomic status (SES). SES has a large effect on individual health. As highlighted in Chapter 7, people with higher SES exhibit better health in a wide variety of settings and for a number of measures of health (Marmot, 1994). Furthermore, SES has changed substantially in recent years. Between 1970 and 1998, for example, the share of the elderly with more than a high school degree rose from 15 percent to 36 percent. Some evidence suggests that increased educational attainment of the elderly can explain part of the reduction in disability (Freedman and Martin, 1999). The existence of these socioeconomic factors in and of themselves does not constitute full explanations, but rather emphasizes the need to better understand the pathways through which they are linked to behavioral, environmental, and psychosocial variables and underlying neurophysiological mechanisms.

A third idea invokes more macro-level influences, namely, the impact of public health measures either in childhood or earlier in adulthood. Many infectious diseases affect health long after a person has passed the infectious stage (Costa, 1998), and there is recent evidence that nutrition as early as the fetal stage affects health in midlife and later (Barker, 1997a, b). Public health advances in the past century thus may have made important contributions to health among the elderly.

Many public health changes may also be linked with macro-level policies, such as the Surgeon General's report on smoking in 1964 (U.S. DHEW, 1964) or prohibitions against smoking in public places. Welfare reform can potentially be associated with health impacts on children. Regulations regarding the geographic placement and protective features of toxic waste dumps can influence the health of entire communities. Analyses of the impact of policies such as these are frequently undertaken by special-interest groups. Monitoring such programs over long periods of time is, however, necessary to establish trends and deviations from them, as illustrated with the case of smoking and its much later disease sequelae (lung cancer, chronic bronchitis and emphysema, cardiovascular diseases; Warner, 2000). An important research priority is support for analyses of the health impacts of these policies. Linking them to the health of communities and of individuals is critically needed.

A final hypothesis concerning improvements in health is that medical advances, in the form of new therapies or prescription drugs, have played a major role. There clearly have been impressive medical advances in the past half century. Consider just one example: the treatment of severe coronary artery disease, which a half-century ago consisted largely of rest, hoping that less strain on the heart would reduce damage from the event. Today, therapy includes acute surgical advances such as cardiac catheterization, bypass surgery, and angioplasty; acute medical interventions such as thrombolysis; and less acute pharmaceutical innovations such as oral diuretics, beta blockers, ACE inhibitors, and calcium channel blockers. These advances have certainly contributed to reduced mortality and probably to reduced morbidity as well (Cutler et al., 1998).

Our ability to empirically differentiate among these various explanations of improved health outcomes has been significantly enhanced by recent developments in data sources. The availability of information from medical claims for large numbers of patients is one such advance. A decade ago medical records on representative groups of patients with particular conditions were not available. Today, Medicare and many private medical insurers in the United States keep such information and use it for this type of research. A second advance has been the implementation of longitudinal population surveys collecting information on socioeconomic status, early life resources, work conditions, family stress and support, physical and mental health, and medical care received that are also linked to earnings records from Social Security systems and medical care utilization from health insurers. Longitudinal data are essential because changing disability will be fully understood only by following the same people over time. The National Long-Term Care Survey, Health and Retirement Study (HRS), and Asset and Health Dynamics Survey (AHEAD) are three recent data sets having information that will be enormously important in this research. Other data sets could be designed (or relevant questions appended to existing surveys) to allow even more valuable research.

Communicable Diseases

The spread of STDs is influenced by three factors: (1) the average risk of infection per exposure, (2) the average rate of sexual partner change within the population, (3) and the average duration of the infectious period. The average duration of infection depends largely on availability and use of medical treatments. Medical treatment for STDs is generally poor in the United States (Holmes, 1994), with some evidence suggesting that overall lack of funding limits the ability of people to receive treatment.

Behavioral changes affecting the rate of sexual partner change are a second explanation for rising STD rates. The age of first sexual intercourse has been falling, rates of unsafe sex are rising, and the number of partners is increasing. The behavioral factors underlying these changes are less clear. One factor may be changes in social norms about appropriate sexual behavior. But other factors include economic circumstances such as the proportion of women working, physical circumstances such as the mix of rich and poor within cities, amount of crowding, and social programs such as the size of welfare benefits and the availability of medical treatments.

Understanding these behavioral and social determinants is central to reducing the spread of STDs. As emphasized in Chapter 6, the relation between community variables and individual behavior is an extremely fruitful area for behavioral and social science research. Work on these areas will be greatly enhanced by ongoing monitoring of STDs and tuberculosis by the CDC. STD and tuberculosis rates can now be measured overall and at the level of particular communities, which will significantly increase our ability to understand the role of community factors in these health outcomes.

Changes in Child Health

Rates of infant mortality and low birth weight are each driven by a confluence of conditions that include low socioeconomic status; poor or no prenatal care; high-risk health behaviors (e.g., smoking, drinking, and drug abuse by pregnant mothers); and chronic exposure to violence, poverty, and nonsupportive social networks. The teen birth rate is strongly correlated with the mother having grown up in an environment in which at least four of the following six conditions held: (1) as a child she was not living with two parents; (2) the household head was a high school dropout; (3) family income was below the poverty line; (4) the parent(s) did not have steady, full-time employment; (5) the family was receiving welfare benefits; and (6) she did not have health insurance (Annie E. Casey Foundation, 1999). All the above conditions vary dramatically by state and by county in the United States. For example, the percentage of children living in families that satisfy four or more of the above high-risk conditions for teen parenthood in 1996 varied from 7 percent in New Hampshire to 21 percent in Mississippi and 39 percent in the District of Columbia.

A more subtle understanding of pathways to low-birth-weight babies, teen parenthood, and infant mortality requires multilevel analyses linking community characteristics with individual histories. Much remains to be done in this area. The recent methodological advances and recommended research priorities for Chapter 6 can be expected to play a central role in future developments.

Turning to asthma, the most common chronic disease of childhood, a deep understanding of its causes still lies in the future. Several current National Institutes of Health (NIH) initiatives are aimed at addressing this knowledge gap. The National Heart, Lung, and Blood Institute (NHLBI) has an initiative aimed at specifying how genetic and environmental factors interact in the developing lung and lead to the onset of asthma. One study sponsored by NHLBI will examine the cellular and molecular mechanisms underlying asthma's relationship with sleep and day-night events. The National Institute of Environmental Health Sciences (NIEHS) has a new Environmental Genome Project that will study different populations in different parts of the country in order to examine how interaction between the environment and certain genes leads to diseases like asthma. The National Institute of Allergy and Infectious Diseases (NIAID) and NIEHS are extending the Inner City Asthma Study, a study of children with asthma in seven U.S. cities that is examining the effects of interventions to reduce children's exposure to indoor allergens and improve communication with their primary care physicians. This investigation also involves collaboration with the Environmental Protection Agency to evaluate the effects of exposure to indoor and outdoor pollutants. Integrating findings from these studies into a unified multilevel explanation of how asthma comes about, together with an assessment of preventive and curative interventions is an important future priority that will require integrative analyses of the sort described throughout this report.

HEALTH AND THE MACROECONOMY

The health status of the population may have macroeconomic effects in addition to affecting individual behavior. Empirically, countries that are less healthy are poorer than countries that are more healthy, and their incomes grow less rapidly. Thus, the income gap between more and less healthy countries is increasing over time. Recent research indicates that life expectancy is a powerful predictor of national income levels and subsequent economic growth (Fogel, 1999). Studies consistently find a strong effect of health on growth rates. Economic historians have concluded that perhaps 30 percent of the estimated per capita growth rate in Britain between 1780 and 1979 was a result of improvements in health and nutritional status (Fogel and Costa, 1997). That lies within the range of estimates produced by cross-country studies using data from the last 30-40 years (Jamison et al., 1998).

Health improvements also influence economic growth through their impact on demography. For example, in the 1940s rapid health improvements in East Asia provided a catalyst for demographic transition. An initial decline in infant and child mortality first dramatically increased the number of young people and then somewhat later prompted a fall in fertility rates. These asynchronous changes in mortality and fertility, which comprise the first phase of what is called the "demographic transition," substantially altered East Asia's age distribution. After a time lag the working-age population began growing much faster than young dependents, temporarily creating a disproportionately high percentage of working-age adults. This bulge in the age structure of the population created an opportunity for increased economic growth (Bloom, 1999).

Over the past several years, the Pan American Health Organization/ Inter-American Development Bank and the United Nations Economic Commission for Latin America and the Caribbean carried out a study to elucidate relations between investments in health, economic growth, and household productivity (WHO, 1999). Estimates based on data from Mexico throw some light on the time frame in which health affects economic indicators. High life expectancy at birth for males and females has an economic impact 0-5 years later. The impact of male life expectancy on the economy appears to be greater than that of female life expectancy, possibly because of the higher level of economic activity among males. The data suggest that for each additional year of life expectancy there will be an additional 1 percent increase in gross domestic product 15 years later. Similar findings were found for schooling.

Studies of this kind are in their infancy compared to other studies described in this report. Much remains to be done to link macro-level associations to the community and individual-level dynamics as discussed in Chapters 2, 3, 5, and 6. Understanding the reciprocal relationships between population health and the macroeconomy and their linkages to micro-level behavioral dynamics and intermediate-level community and social structural influences is a high-priority research direction. Indeed, it is precisely results such as those for Mexico, described above, that have implications for national economic policies leading to sustained commitments to investments in health. Providing clear evidence about linkages to community and individual levels can substantially strengthen the arguments for national commitments.

Health and the economy have long been linked by the practice of having children to ensure being cared for in old age. This is still true in many countries, but with public-sector innovations such as Social Security and medical care, the direct need for children as insurance has declined. In its place are issues of individual behavior (whether people live alone or with their children, whether they work or retire) and social questions about whether society can afford to provide care to an aging population.

The backdrop for much of the concern about changes in health is the strain that increasing length of life places on public programs in industrialized countries. The Social Security system in the United States is forecast to become insolvent around 2030, and Medicare is expected to be insolvent long before then. This situation, repeated throughout the developed world and in many developing countries, is made worse as population growth rates fall. Health improvements have hidden costs if they lead to difficulty financing public-sector programs for the elderly. However, recent evidence of rectangularization of survival curves, not only for mortality but for the age-specific onset of disability and chronic diseases (Vita et al., 1998), suggests that prevention strategies may be having positive countervailing effects.

Health improvements can play a substantial role in solving public-sector problems. People who develop a serious illness late in their working life are more likely to retire early than are people who do not experience a serious illness at that age (Smith, 1999), which reduces their lifetime earnings. Adolescents who are diagnosed with depression are less likely to get a college degree than are those not so diagnosed (Berndt et al., 2000) and thus are likley to earn less over their lifetime. Advances in interventions that alleviate these health burdens could substantially reduce the public-sector financial burden. In any case, a central economic challenge facing the public sector is how to prepare for an aging society.

THE HEALTH CARE SYSTEM

The medical system is an important part of health. Indeed, public discussion about health focuses to an overwhelming degree on access to medical care. Understanding how the system operates and how well it works is therefore a central issue for behavioral and social research. We address three issues of concern in current and future evaluations of the health care system: (1) the effects of medical care on improving health, (2) the managed care debate, and (3) growing public interest in alternative medicine.

Effectiveness of Medical Care

Research shows mixed results regarding the value of the medical system. We illustrate these issues with medical care for the elderly, but the same issues apply to those who are not elderly, for example, asthma in children or disease transmission in teens and young adults. Some research highlights the positive effect of medical care on improving health. As noted above, one of the leading theories for reduced disability among the elderly is that such advances result from medical technology improvements. This view is widespread among biomedical researchers: medical advances, they believe, embodied in new technologies lead to significant health gains. Other research, however, highlights the apparently low return from additional medical spending. For example, Medicare spending varies by a factor of two among areas of the country, with no apparent differences in health outcomes (CECS, 1998). Research on heart attack patients shows that intensive procedures are used up to five times more frequently in the United States than in Canada, but mortality rates are the same in the two countries (Rouleau et al., 1993; Mark et al., 1994; Tu et al., 1997). Indeed, within the United States, people who live close to high-tech hospitals receive intensive services more frequently than people who live farther away from such hospitals, but again health outcomes are essentially the same (McClellan et al., 1994). The value of additional medical spending is therefore unclear and is a needed avenue for future research.

Several explanations have been proposed for the disparate or conflicting findings about whether medical care has high or relatively low returns. One hypothesis is that medical care is valuable but is often applied inappropriately. For example, areas that spend a lot on medical care may simply give the technology to more people than will benefit from it. Much evidence supports the view that medical care is frequently wasted. Studies of medical procedure use in the United States, for example, find that a significant number of patients receiving high-tech services should not receive them on the basis of published clinical studies (Chassin et al., 1987; Winslow et al., 1988a, b; Greenspan et al., 1988). Other evidence is less supportive, however, finding that rates of inappropriate procedure use are no greater in areas with high usage rates compared to areas with lower usage rates. Reconciling conflicting evidence about the value of medical care is an important priority for future research.

It also has been proposed that preventive care is used in inverse proportion to more intensive medical services, so that people not receiving intensive treatment still have good outcomes. This is claimed to explain the lack of outcome differences between the United States and Canada. Canada has more complete coverage for outpatient pharmaceuticals than does the United States. Increased use of pharmaceuticals may allow Canadians to live longer, offsetting the survival advantage that comes from more intensive procedure use in the United States.

The distinction between over-time and point-in-time analysis must also be considered in evaluating the effectiveness of medical care. Many studies that find that medical care has a high rate of return compare treatments at different points in time, that is, before and after a particular technology is available. For example, changes in the treatment of heart attacks during the 1980s are associated with large increases in survival (Cutler and Sheiner, 1998). The same is true for care of low-birth-weight infants between 1950 and 1990 (Cutler and Meara, 2000). In contrast, studies that find that medical care has a low rate of return generally look at the use of the same treatment in different localities at the same point in time. Differences in use at a point in time may be more wasteful than increased use over time.

An increasing number of cost-effectiveness analyses of preventive strategies and alternative therapies are appearing. For example, Trussell et al. (1997) analyzed the economic benefits of adolescent contraceptive use utilizing information from a national private payer data base and from the California Medicaid program. Their study estimated the costs of acquiring and using 11 contraceptive methods appropriate for adolescents, treating associated side effects, providing medical care related to an unintended pregnancy during contraceptive use, and treating sexually transmitted diseases (STDs) and compared them with the costs of not using a contraceptive method. The average annual cost per adolescent at risk of unintended pregnancy who uses no method of contraception is $1,267 ($1,079 for unintended pregnancy and $188 for STDs) in the private sector and $677 ($541 for unintended pregnancy and $137 for STDs) in the public sector. After one year of use private-sector savings from adolescent contraceptive use ranged from $308 for an implant designed to prevent ovulation to $946 for the male condom. Public-sector savings rose from $60 for the implant to $525 for the male condom. Both the use of male condoms with another method and the advance provision of backup emergency contraceptive pills provided additional savings.

Shifting to an example of the cost effectiveness of cholesterol-lowering therapies, Prosser et al. (2000) found that ratios varied according to different risk factors. Specifically, incremental cost effectiveness ratios were found for primary prevention with a low fat, low cholesterol diet (National Cholesterol Education Program step I), ranging from $1,900 per quality-adjusted life-year (QALY) gained to $500,000 per QALY depending on risk subgroup characteristics. Primary prevention with a statin (a cholesterol-lowering drug) compared with diet therapy was $54,000 per QALY to $1.4 million per QALY. Secondary prevention with a statin cost less than $50,000 per QALY for all risk subgroups. Primary prevention with a step I diet seems to be cost effective for most risk subgroups defined by age, sex, and the presence of additional risk factors. It may not be cost effective for otherwise healthy young women. In addition, primary prevention with a statin may not be cost effective for younger men and women with few risk factors, given the option of secondary prevention and of primary prevention in older age groups. Secondary prevention with a statin seems to be cost effective for all risk subgroups and is cost saving for some high-risk subgroups.

As a further illustration, an economic evaluation was conducted alongside a randomized controlled trial of two lifestyle interventions (e.g., education and video to assess risk factors, program plan for risk factor behavior change) and a routine care (control) group to assess cost effectiveness for patients with risk factors for cardiovascular disease (Salkeld et al., 1997). The cost per QALY for males ranged from $152,000 to $204,000. Further analysis suggested that a program targeted at high-risk males would cost $30,000 per QALY. The lifestyle interventions had no significant effect on cardiovascular risk factors when compared to routine patient care. There remains insufficient evidence that lifestyle programs conducted in general practice are effective. Resources for general-practice-based lifestyle programs may be better spent on high-risk patients who are contemplating changes in risk factor behaviors. Alternatively, the extensive literature on the economics of coronary heart disease prevention (Brown and Garber, 1998) suggests that many programs (e.g., exercise, smoking cessation, detection and treatment of hypertension, cholesterol reduction) are highly cost effective.

While these examples are illustrative of the kinds of studies needed on a wider scale, it is important to underscore that such inquiries can have substantial impact on the quality of care provided by a diverse range of practitioners. In addition, errors in specification of therapeutic programs, mistakes made during surgical procedures, improper diagnoses, and faulty laboratory procedures are being documented on an increasingly broad scale. Such lines of inquiry are important for understanding the behavior of health care providers as a function of economic and organizational constraints placed on them. It will be equally important to turn solid research findings into improved practices. This will require effective communication and ongoing dialogue between the research community and practitioners. Cultural factors also play a prominent role here, since patients of different ethnic backgrounds approach—or do not approach—health care providers with very diverse views of health and wellness (Kleinman, 1981, 1989). Also important for the future will be analyses of data on medical treatments matched to health outcomes. Such data are now becoming widely available through Medicare and large insurers.

The Managed Care Debate

Public concern about managed care is intense, as recent legislative efforts to enact a patients' bill of rights attest. Research about how managed care actually affects medical practice, however, is limited. Changes in insurance coverage for nonelderly Americans between 1980 and 1996 were dramatic. In 1980, 92 percent of the population had traditional indemnity insurance, with 8 percent in health maintenance organizations (HMOs). In 1996 only 3 percent of the population remained in unmanaged fee-for-service plans. An additional 22 percent were in managed fee-for-service plans. The bulk of the population was enrolled in various types of managed care programs, including traditional HMOs, preferred-provider organizations (PPOs), and point-of-service plans (POSs). The spread of managed care is largely responsible for the reduced rate of growth of medical spending in the 1990s (Cutler and Sheiner, 1998).

This trend has provoked fundamental questions. How does managed care save money: by restricting the number of services provided or by cutting payments for services? That is, managed care might affect the delivery of medical care in two ways: by altering the access rules (determining which people have access to medical providers) and the payment rules (determining reimbursement to providers). People with managed care insurance typically have more restrictive access to providers and high-tech care than do people in traditional indemnity insurance. On the other hand, people with managed care insurance generally have lower costs than do those with indemnity insurance.

The central issue is how health outcomes are affected by managed care. A second issue is whether the rise of managed care affects the diffusion of medical technology and whether that will be good or bad. Understanding the full incentives of managed care is difficult and requires the participation of both economic and medical expertise, for example, in understanding exactly how physicians are paid and what services they are able to provide. Sociological and psychological input is necessary as well. For example, physicians treated as employees of a managed care insurer may behave differently than physicians who see themselves as running their own practice. The degree to which managed care affects physician practice may depend on how it changes physicians' perceptions of their role in the medical system as much as it changes their actual ability to provide certain services. Research has yet to explore this issue.

Managed care might also have a direct effect on the extent to which providers acquire and use particular technologies. Several recent papers argue that managed care has reduced the diffusion of hospital-based technologies, including diagnostic scanners and some surgical procedures (Cutler and Sheiner, 1998; Baker and Spetz, 1999). If such changes in access translate into change in utilization, it could have important implications for the long-term value of the medical sector. Research on this issue is just beginning as well.

In summary, the phenomenal change in the medical system encompassed by managed care, coupled with the availability of rich sources of data, make this topic a prime candidate for future research. Understanding the economic and health consequences of managed care has great import for informing public policy pertaining to the health care system.

Alternative Medicine Therapies

A large and expanding component of the U.S. health care system involves alternative medicine therapies, functionally defined as interventions neither taught widely in medical schools nor generally available in U.S. hospitals (Eisenberg et al., 1993). In 1990 a national survey of alternative medicine prevalence, costs, and patterns of use demonstrated that alternative medicine has a substantial presence in the U.S. health care system. Since that time, an increasing number of insurers and managed care organizations have offered alternative medicine programs and benefits. Correlatively, the majority of U.S. medical schools now offer courses on alternative medicine (Wetzel et al., 1998; Eisenberg et al., 1998).

In a follow-up national survey conducted in 1997 (Eisenberg et al., 1998), data were assembled that allowed for quantitative assessment of trends in alternative medicine use over that time period. Use of at least one of 16 alternative therapies investigated increased from 8 percent in 1990 to 42.1 percent in 1997. The therapies increasing the most included herbal medicine, massage, megavitamins, self-help groups, folk remedies, energy healing, and homeopathy. In both the 1990 and 1997 surveys alternative therapies were used most frequently for chronic conditions, including back problems, anxiety, depression, and headaches. The percentage of users paying entirely out of pocket for services provided by alternative medicine practitioners did not change significantly between 1990 (64.0 percent) and 1997 (58.3 percent). Extrapolations to the U.S. population suggest a 47.3 percent increase in total visits to alternative medicine practitioners, from 427 million in 1990 to 629 million in 1997, thereby exceeding total visits to all U.S. primary care physicians. An estimated 15 million adults in 1997 took prescription medications concurrently with herbal remedies and/or high-dose vitamins (18.4 percent of all prescription users). Estimated expenditures for alternative medicine professional services increased 45.2 percent between 1990 and 1997 and were conservatively estimated at $21.2 billion in 1997, with at least $12.2 billion paid out of pocket. This exceeds the 1997 out-of-pocket expenditures for all U.S. hospitalizations. Total 1997 out-of-pocket expenditures relating to alternative therapies were conservatively estimated at $27 billion, which is comparable to the projected 1997 out-of-pocket expenditures for all U.S. physician services.

The large economic impact of alternative medicine clearly demands research attention. Specifically, substantial resources should be devoted to clinical and integrated biological and social science research to provide rigorous understanding of the role of these interventions in the health of the U.S. population. This is important for establishing the credibility of claims for alternative medicine therapies. Part of this line of inquiry should include research on why placebos sometimes work and for whom. More generally, the broad area of mind/body relationships and their neurobiological underpinnings represent a vast research opportunity for the future. A useful example of the kind of knowledge development and synthesis that are needed is the elaborate study of meditation and neurobiology by Austin (1998). The new NIH trans-institute initiative that recently established five mind/body centers around the United States constitutes a further important step in this direction.

FUTURE DIRECTIONS IN POPULATION SURVEYS

Several sources of data and methodologies will be essential in addressing the agendas described above. Perhaps the most basic need is for enhanced longitudinal population-level surveys. Such surveys should be enhanced in three ways:

1. They need to be linked to administrative records on the receipt of medical care and on work histories. Such linkage is vital because individuals will not recall all of the medical care they have received nor their earnings records.

2. Surveys need to be supplemented with community-level variables to determine how the social and economic environments affect individual behavior.

3. They need to have basic biological markers. Incorporating indicators of cumulative physiological risk (e.g., allostatic load) as standard components of longitudinal survey protocols would provide a basis for the integrative analyses recommended throughout this report. Augmenting longitudinal surveys with physical health examinations would be of enormous value, as the Framingham Study has shown.

Data from medical systems are also essential. Health insurers in the United States and other countries have access to unparalleled data on medical treatments and outcomes. These data can be used to study the value of the medical system. They can also address questions about behavior and community-level variables because they often contain detailed information on health conditions and medical treatments at the community level. Finally, we stress the role for international comparative work in answering the full range of population health questions discussed in this chapter. Economic, social, and medical systems differ greatly across countries, and thus international work is a natural laboratory for analysis.

RECOMMENDATIONS

We urge NIH to invest new resources in research to identify linkages between population health trends and the behavioral, environmental, and psychosocial factors emphasized in preceding chapters. Priority should be given to the following topics:

• multilevel analyses necessary to advance rigorous explanations for the observed dynamics of the health of populations, giving particular emphasis to behavioral risk and protective factors and to psychosocial and environmental influences on aggregate-level health changes;

• development of projection methodologies to provide defensible scenarios of how health changes will affect society in the future;

• continue and expand multi-institute support of research on child health, particularly asthma and its costs, both economic (e.g., parental absence from work) and social (e.g., family burden, child development);

• increase support for research on the reciprocal relationships between population health and the macroeconomy, together with linkages to community and individual-level dynamics as discussed in prior chapters;

• develop new initiatives to investigate the conflicting findings about whether medical care has high or low returns for whom, when, and how. Importantly, data on medical treatments must be matched to health outcomes;

• increase support for research on the economic and health costs or benefits of managed care (of central importance are studies that clarify how health outcomes are affected by managed care);

• establish new trans-institute priorities to evaluate the effectiveness of alternative medicine therapies as well as to clarify their economic impact.

REFERENCES

Annie E. Casey Foundation. 1999 *Kids Count Data Book, 1999* (Baltimore: Annie E. Casey Foundation).

Austin J. 1998 *Zen and the Brain* (Cambridge MA: MIT Press).

Baker L, Spetz J. 1999 "Managed care and medical technology growth" NBER Working Paper 6894 (Cambridge MA: National Bureau of Economic Research).

Barker DJ. 1997a "The fetal origins of coronary heart disease" *Acta Paediatrica* 422/suppl.:78-82.

Barker DJ. 1997b "Maternal nutrition, fetal nutrition and disease in later life" *Nutrition* 13/9:807-13.

Berndt ER, Koran LM, Finkelstein SN, Gelenberg AJ, Kornstein SG, Miller IW, Thase ME, Trapp GM, Keller MB. 2000 "Lost human capital from early-onset chronic depression" *American Journal of Psychiatry* 157/6:940-947.

Bloom BR. 1999 "The future of public health" *Nature* 402/suppl. 2 December:C63-C64.

Brown AD, Garber AM. 1998 "Cost effectiveness of coronary heart disease prevention strategies in adults" *Pharmacoeconomics* 14/1:27-48.

CECS (Center for Evaluative Clinical Sciences), Dartmouth Medical School. 1998 *Dartmouth Atlas of Health Care* (Chicago: American Hospital Publishing).

CDC (Centers for Disease Control and Prevention). 1999a "Progress toward the elimination of tuberculosis—United States, 1998" *Morbidity and Mortality Weekly Report* 48/33:732-736.

CDC (Centers for Disease Control and Prevention). 1999b *Tracking the Hidden Epidemics: Trends in the STD Epidemics in the United States* (Atlanta: Centers for Disease Control and Prevention).

CDC (Centers for Disease Control and Prevention). 1999c "Cigarette smoking among adults—United States, 1997" *MMWR Morbidity and Mortality Weekly Report* 48:993-996.

CDC (Centers for Disease Control and Prevention). 1999d *Reported Tuberculosis in the United States, 1998* (Atlanta: Centers for Disease Control and Prevention).

Chassin MR, Kosecoff J, Park RE, Winslow CM, Kahn KL, Merrick NJ, Keesey J, Fink A, Solomon DH, Brook RH. 1987 "Does inappropriate use explain geographic variations in the use of health care services? A study of three procedures" *Journal of the American Medical Association* 258/18:2533-2537.

Costa DL. 1998 "Understanding the twentieth century decline in chronic conditions among older men" Working Paper 6859 (Cambridge MA: National Bureau of Economic Research).

Cutler D, Meara E. 2000 "The technology of birth: Is it worth it?" in Garber A (ed.). *Frontiers in Health Policy Research, Volume III* (Cambridge MA: MIT Press).

Cutler DM, Sheiner L. 1998 "Managed care and the growth of medical expenditures" in Garber A (ed.). *Frontiers in Health Policy Research, Volume I* (Cambridge MA: MIT Press).

Cutler DM, McClellan M, Remler D, Newhouse JP. 1998 "Are medical prices declining? Evidence from heart attack treatments" *Quarterly Journal of Economics* 133/4:991-1024.

Daszak P, Cunningham AA, Hyatt AD. 2000 "Emerging infectious diseases of wildlife—Threats to biodiversity and human health" *Science* 287/5452:443-449.

Eisenberg DM, Kessler RC, Foster C, Norlock FE, Calkins DR, Delbanco TL. 1993 "Unconventional medicine in the United States: Prevalence, costs, and patterns of use" *New England Journal of Medicine* 328/4:246-252.

Eisenberg DM, Davis RB, Ettner SL, Appel S, Wilkey S, Van Rompay M, Kessler RC. 1998 "Trends in alternative medicine use in the United States, 1990-1997: Results of a follow-up national survey" *Journal of the American Medical Association* 280/18:1569-1575.

Eng TR, Butler WT. 1997 *The Hidden Epidemic: Confronting Sexually Transmitted Diseases* (Washington DC: National Academy Press).

Fogel RW. 1999 "Catching up with the Economy" *The American Economic Review* 89/1:1-21.

Fogel RW, Costa DL. 1997 "A theory of technophysio evolution, with some implications for forecasting population, health care costs, and pension costs" *Demography* 34/1:49-66.

Freedman VA, Martin LG. 1998 "Understanding trends in functional limitations among older Americans" *American Journal of Public Health* 88/10:1457-1462.

Freedman VA, Martin LG. 1999 "The role of education in explaining and forecasting trends in functional limitations among older Americans" *Demography* 36/4:461-473.

Greenspan AM, Kay HR, Berger BC, Greenberg RM, Greenspon AJ, Gaughan MJ. 1988 "Incidence of unwarranted implantation of permanent cardiac pacemakers in a large medical population" *New England Journal of Medicine* 318/13:158-163.

Hill JO, Peters JC. 1998 "Environmental contributions to the obesity epidemic" *Science* 280:1371-1374.

Holmberg SD. 1996 "The estimated prevalence and incidence of HIV in 96 large US metropolitan areas" *American Journal of Public Health* 86/5:642-654.

Holmes KK. 1994 "Human ecology and behavior and sexually transmitted bacterial infections" *Proceedings of the National Academy of Sciences of the United States of America* 91/7:2448-2455.

Jacobzone S. 2000 "Coping with aging: International challenges" *Health Affairs* 19/3:213-225.

Jamison DT, Lau LJ, Wang J. 1998 "Health's contribution to economic growth, 1965-1990" in *Health, Health Policy and Economic Outcomes: Final Report Health and Development Satellite, WHO Director-General Transition Team* (Geneva: World Health Organization):61-80.

Kaiser Family Foundation. 1998 *Sexually Transmitted Diseases in America: How Many Cases and at What Cost?* (Menlo Park: Kaiser Family Foundation).

Kleinman A. 1981 *Patients and Healers in the Context of Culture* (Berkeley: University of California Press).

Kleinman A. 1989 *The Illness Narratives: Suffering, Healing, and the Human Condition.* (New York: Basic Books).

Lederberg J, Shope RE, Oakes SC Jr. (eds.). 1992 *Emerging Infections: Microbial Threats to Health in the United States* (Washington DC: National Academy Press).

Lee I, Paffenbarger RS, Hsieh C. 1991 "Physical activity and risk of developing colorectal cancer among college alumni" *Journal of National Cancer Institute* 83:1324-1329.

Manson JE, Tosteson H, Ridker PM, Satterfield S, Hebert P, O'Connor GT, Buring JE, Hennekens CH. 1992 "The primary prevention of myocardial infarction" *New England Journal of Medicine* 326/21:1406-1416.

Manton KG, Corder L, Stallard E. 1997 "Chronic disability trends in elderly United States populations: 1982-1994" *Proceedings of the National Academy of Sciences of the United States of America* 94/6:2593-2598.

Mark DB, Naylor CD, Hlatky MA, Califf RM, Topol EJ, Granger CB, Knight JD, Nelson CL, Lee KL, Clapp-Channing NE, Sutherland W, Pilote L, Armstrong PW. 1994 "Use of medical resources and quality of life after acute myocardial infarction in Canada and the United States" *New England Journal of Medicine* 331/17:1130-1135.

Marmot MG. 1994 "Social differentials in health within and between populations" *Daedalus* 123/4:197-216.

Marmot MG, Smith GD, Stansfield S, Patel C, North F, Head J, White I, Brunner E, Feeney A. 1991 "Health inequalities among British civil servants: The Whitehall II Study" *Lancet* 337/8754:1387-1393.

McClellan M, McNeil BJ, Newhouse JP. 1994 "Does more intensive treatment of acute myocardial infarction in the elderly reduce mortality? Analysis using instrumental variables" *Journal of the American Medical Association* 272/11:859-866.

McGinnis JM, Foege WH. 1993 "Actual causes of death in the United States" *Journal of the American Medical Association* 270/18:2207-2212.

Melin B, Lundberg U. 1997 "A biopsychosocial approach to work-stress and musculoskeletal disorders" *Journal of Psychophysiology* 11/3:238-247.

Mendez D, Warner KE. 1998 "Has smoking cessation ceased? Expected trends in the prevalence of smoking in the United States" *American Journal of Epidemiology* 148:249-258.

Mokdad A, Serdula MK, Dietz WH, Bowman BA, Marks JS, Koplan JP. 1999 "The spread of the obesity epidemic in the United States" *Journal of the American Medical Association* 282:1519-1522.

Murray CJ, Salomon JA. 1998 "Modeling the impact of global tuberculosis control strategies" *Proceedings of the National Academy of Sciences of the United States of America* 95/23:13881-13886.

NCHS (National Center for Health Statistics). 1982, 1984, 1987, 1990, 1992, 1993 *Current Estimates from the National Health Interview Survey* Series 10, Nos. 150, 156, 166, 181, 189, and 190 (Hyattsville, MD: U.S. Department of Health and Human Services).

Paffenbarger RS, Hyde RT, Wing AL. 1990 "Physical activity and physical fitness as determinants of health and longevity" in Bouchard C, Shephard RJ, Stephens T, Sutton JR, McPherson BD (eds.). *Exercise, Fitness, and Health* (Champaign IL: Human Kinetics Books).

Perutz M. 1998 "Centenarians. And they all lived happily ever after" *Economist* Feb 7:82-83.

Prosser LA, Stinnett AA, Goldman PA, Williams LW, Hunink MG, Goldman L, Weinstein MC. 2000 "Cost-effectiveness of cholesterol-lowering therapies according to selected patient characteristics" *Annals of Internal Medicine* 132(10):769-779.

Rose G. 1992 *The Strategy of Preventive Medicine* (Oxford U.K.: Oxford University Press).

Rosenberg PS. 1995 "Scope of the AIDS epidemic in the United States" *Science* 270/5240:1372-1375.

Rouleau JL, Moye LA, Pfeffer MA, Arnold JM, Bernstein V, Cuddy TE, Dagenais GR, Geltman EM, Goldman S, Gordon D, Hamm P, Klein M, Lamas GA, McCans J, McEwan P, Menapace FJ, Parker JO, Sestier F, Sussex B, Braunwald E. 1993 "A comparison of management patterns after acute myocardial infarction in Canada and the United States" *New England Journal of Medicine* 328/11:779-784.

Salkeld G, Phongsavan P, Oldenberg B, Johanneson M, Convery P, Graham-Clarke P, Walker S, Shaw J. 1997 "The cost-effectiveness of a cardiovascular risk reduction program in general practice" *Health Policy* 41/2:105-119.

Singer BH, Manton KG. 1998 "The effects of health changes on projections of health service needs for the elderly population of the United States" *Proceedings of the National Academy of Sciences of the United States of America* 95/26:15618-15622.

Smith JP. 1999 "Healthy bodies and thick wallets: The dual relation between health and economic status" *The Journal of Economic Perspectives* 13/2:145-166.

Tauber G. 1998 "As obesity rates rise, experts struggle to explain why" *Science* 280:1367-1368.

Trussell J, Koenig J, Stewart F, Darroch J. 1997 "Medical care cost savings from adolescent contraceptive use" *Family Planning Perspectives* 29:248-263.

Tu JV, Pashos CL, Naylor CD, Chen E, Normand SL, Newhouse JP, McNeil BJ. 1997 "Use of cardiac procedures and outcomes in elderly patients with myocardial infarction in the United States and Canada" *New England Journal of Medicine* 336/21:1500-1505.

UNAIDS. 1998 *The UNAIDS Report* (Geneva: UNAIDS).

U.S. DHEW (U.S. Department of Health, Education, and Welfare). 1964 *Smoking and Health.* Report of the Advisory Committee to the Surgeon General of the Public Health Service. PHS Publication No. 1103 (Washington DC: U.S. Department of Health, Education, and Welfare).

U.S. DHHS (U.S. Department of Health and Human Services). 1988 *The Surgeon General's Report on Nutrition and Health* PHS 88-50210 (Washington DC: Department of Health and Human Services).

U.S. DHHS (U.S. Department of Health and Human Services). 1989 *Reducing the Health Consequences of Smoking: 25 Years of Progress* DHHS No.(CDC) 89-8411 (Washington DC: Department of Health and Human Services).

U.S. DHHS (U.S. Department of Health and Human Services). 1996 *Trends in the Well-Being of America's Children and Youth* (Washington DC: Department of Health and Human Services).

U.S. DHHS (U.S. Department of Health and Human Services). 2000 *Healthy People 2010: Understanding and Improving Health (2 volumes).* (Washington DC: Department of Health and Human Services).

Vita AJ, Terry RB, Hubert HB, Fries JF. 1998 "Aging, health risks, and cumulative disability" *New England Journal of Medicine* 338/15:1035-1041.

Warner KE. 2000 "The need for, and value of, a multi-level approach to disease prevention: The case of tobacco control" in Smedley BD, Syme, SL (eds.). *Promoting Health: Intervention Strategies from Social and Behavioral Research* (Washington DC: National Academy Press) 326-351.

Wetzel MS, Eisenberg DM, Kaptchuk TJ. 1998 "Courses involving complementary and alternative medicine at U.S. medical schools" *Journal of the American Medical Association* 280/9:784-787.

Wickelgren I. 1998 "Obesity: How big a problem?" *Science* 280:1364-1367.

Winslow, CM, Kosecoff JB, Chassin M, Kanouse DE, Brook RH. 1988a "The appropriateness of performing coronary artery bypass surgery" *Journal of the American Medical Association* 260/4:505-509.

Winslow CM, Solomon DH, Chassin MR, Kosecoff J, Merrick NJ, Brook RH. 1988b "The appropriateness of carotid endarterectomy" *New England Journal of Medicine* 318/12:721-727.

WHO (World Health Organization). 1999 *The World Health Report* (Geneva: World Health Organization).

9

Interventions

Over the last several decades, numerous preventive and therapeutic interventions have been introduced with the aim of helping people live longer and improve their overall quality of life. Such programs typically fall into four broad categories (see Compas et al., 1998): (1) interventions designed to decrease health risk behaviors, such as alcohol and substance abuse or smoking, or to increase health-promoting behaviors, such as exercise and following a healthy diet; (2) interventions aimed at facilitating effective coping with chronic or life-threatening diseases and conditions, including cancer, HIV/AIDS, asthma, diabetes, arthritis, and stroke; (3) interventions to help manage specific symptoms or problems, such as chronic headaches, back pain, and abdominal pain; and (4) interventions addressing psychopathologies such as bulimia nervosa, anorexia nervosa, and body dysmorphic disorder.

The first two intervention categories emphasize behavioral and social aspects of illness and will be the principal focus of this section. The majority of research on interventions, moreover, has focused mostly on modifying health-risk behaviors. In this report we describe additional ways that behavioral and social factors can be mobilized to improve health, prevent illness, and enhance quality of life. As research identifies new ways that social and behavioral factors affect health, it creates new targets for intervention research and practice.

Preventive and therapeutic interventions can be directed at different levels. At the individual level, interventions activate internal, or psychological resources possessed by the individual and focus on teaching individual skills or strive to change individual behavior. At the social level, interventions attempt to bring to bear the broader resources deriving from contacts with the individual's family, friends, or social network or to change behavior patterns in family groups. At the organizational level, interventions are implemented in specific settings or units such as work sites or schools and target group change. Interventions at the population level are actions targeted at entire communities, towns, or states. In practice, intervention programs can be directed at one level at a time or can cross levels (Sorenson et al., 1998). Indeed at any one time, for example, public health efforts could promote better diets at the community level, schools could offer heart healthy lunches instead of the current fast food options, and individuals could be advised by their primary care providers to reduce fat in their diets.

Behavioral and social interventions can target either prevention or treatment, although these goals frequently coalesce in practice. For example, altering diet or increasing exercise can prevent the initial onset of cardiovascular problems, improve recovery, and prevent reoccurrence of cardiovascular problems. In general, interventions aimed at altering health risk behaviors have both preventive and treatment effects.

Successful intervention programs function on multiple levels (Sorensen et al., 1998). The benefits of targeting individuals at high risk due to their previous or current behavior, such as heavy cigarette smokers, or to a genetic susceptibility such as that of cholesterolemia, is apparent. However, clinical models that intervene with only high-risk individuals miss the potential for preventing disease by addressing other underlying causes contributing to elevated risk. When underlying causes of illness, such as low socioeconomic status are widely distributed in segments of the population, small changes at the population level are likely to have significant effects on overall population-level health. Indeed, many of the new social risk factors, including poverty and social isolation, are better addressed at the family, organizational, or population level than at the level of the individual. Similarly, when risk, such as widespread physical inactivity and overweight, is widely distributed, small changes at the population level to encourage activity (Chesney et al., 2001) are likely to yield greater improvements in the population-attributable risk than larger changes among a smaller number of high-risk individuals (Velicer et al., 1999).

The success of many health-related activities depends on the decision-making competence of the individuals involved. In their day-to-day lives people need to make good choices about diet and exercise, about the safety of their homes and vehicles, about the management of alcohol and anger, and about how to monitor their health status. When problems arise, they must decide when and how to present themselves to health care professionals as well as which treatments to follow. As practitioners, health care professionals must present options in clear and effective ways and protect patients from unwarranted pressures. Health care professionals must also be responsive to cultural diversity in how to work effectively with individuals in the implementation of intervention programs (Kleinman, 1981, 1989).

EXPERIENCE WITH INTERVENTIONS

The following illustrates a range of individual, family, organizational, and population-level interventions that have been undertaken and is not intended to be a comprehensive review. The intent is first to describe an area, smoking cessation, where extensive work has been done to show the scope of social and behavioral interventions possible. Then, attention will be given to newer areas of intervention that show promise. Social and behavioral efforts to prevent smoking initiation or promote cessation have been studied for several decades (Warner, 2000). Extensive reviews document the success of these programs at the individual, school, and community or population levels.

Individual Interventions

Smoking prevention and cessation research illustrates a domain in which multilevel approaches (Warner, 2000) have been particularly effective. Extensive programs for children and teens have tried to prevent youth initiation of tobacco use through school education and counteradvertising campaigns in the media (U.S. DHHS, 1994). A meta-analysis of school interventions aimed at reducing smoking found that effect sizes were largest for interventions that focus on social reinforcement for the target behavior, moderate for those with either a developmental orientation or a focus on changing social norms as a way to influence the target behavior, and small for interventions with a health education focus (Bruvold, 1993). The effect of price increases (taxes) has also been shown to discourage youth smoking (see subsequent section, "Organization- and Population-Level Interventions").

With regard to adult smoking cessation, individual-level programs combining behavioral strategies for quitting with such pharmacological agents as nicotine patches continue to be at the forefront of research and practice. A challenge to these interventions has been maintenance of the positive changes that have been observed following initial training programs (Compas et al., 1998). Smoking cessation is an area that has not only experienced this challenge but where studies to identify effective strategies have been conducted. For example, one study examined alternative maintenance strategies in 744 adults from a health maintenance organization smoking cessation program (Stevens and Hollis, 1989). Participants who achieved smoking cessation (79 percent) were randomly assigned to relapse prevention skills training, group discussion, or no further treatment. Group discussion and no-further-treatment conditions were equivalent in effectiveness (34 percent and 33 percent abstinence after one year), while the skills-training group was significantly superior (41 percent). Further efforts are needed to determine maximally effective strategies to maintain behavior change.

Formal cessation programs commonly succeed in helping 15-25 percent of participants to quit (U.S. DHHS, 1996; Warner, 2000), a figure dramatically higher than all other tobacco control interventions. Nonetheless, it is the case that relatively few smokers participate in these programs, and the vast majority of smokers who quit do so without the aid of a formal program.

Like smoking cessation, there is a portfolio of interventions designed to change other risk behaviors, including diet, physical inactivity, and alcohol and substance use. Many of these interventions are important both to prevent illness in the healthy and to prevent recurrence or delay illness progression in those who are managing chronic illness, such as coronary heart disease. This brings us to the second category of behavioral interventions, involving coping with chronic illness. This is a particularly important area, given the growing segment of the population that lives with chronic illness. Psychological interventions have shown considerable promise in the management of cancer. These interventions have been shown to help individuals manage the side effects of chemotherapy, and there is also evidence that psychosocial interventions can increase disease-free intervals and length of survival for cancer patients (Compas et al., 1998). Moreover, short-term psychiatric group intervention was associated with long-term changes in the natural killer cell (NK) system in a group of patients with newly diagnosed melanoma and good prognoses (Fawzy et al., 1990). At six months, 100 percent of the intervention group showed increases in CD 16 NK cells, 74 percent showed increases in CD 56 NK cells, and 94 percent showed increases in Leu-7 large granular lymphocytes. These changes indicate a consistent increase in the number of NK cells, seemingly in response to the intervention, suggesting that the NK cells' system might be responsive to psychological or behavioral influences. It remains to be determined whether these perturbations in cell immunity have downstream health consequences.

Some evidence supports the effectiveness of social interventions for prolonging survival of cancer patients. One study assessing the effect of group therapy on patients with metastatic breast cancer, for example, found that those participating in weekly group therapy for a year not only experienced reduced anxiety, depression, and pain but survived significantly longer than did controls—by an average of nearly 18 months, measured at a 10-year follow-up (Spiegel et al., 1989). However, other studies have not found positive results. Another study assessing the effect of several types of "supportive" group therapy on breast cancer patients observed no measurable psychological benefit of participation in the group programs compared to routine control care and found no significant difference in survival time (Gellert et al., 1993). It is unlikely that an intervention failing to provide psychological benefit would yield survival advantage.

Effective psychosocial treatments aimed at pain management not only recognize the importance of biological factors but also emphasize the influences that psychological factors (e.g., anxiety, depression, perceived control) and social factors (e.g., family and work environments) can have on the experience of pain (Compas et al., 1998). Several approaches (e.g., cognitive behavioral therapy, operant behavioral therapy, and biofeedback training) have proven efficacious for managing rheumatic diseases, chronic pain syndrome and low back pain, migraine headaches, and irritable bowel syndrome. Considerable evidence supports the effectiveness of cognitive behavioral therapy for reducing bulimia nervosa, showing roughly 80 percent reduction in binge-purge episodes and 50 to 60 percent of patients achieving complete remission (Craighead and Agras, 1991).

Medically prescribed and supervised physical activity forms the keystone of cardiac rehabilitation, and regular exercise by patients with coronary artery disease is associated with reductions in mortality from all cardiovascular causes except sudden death (Naughton, 1992). The addition of psychosocial treatments to standard cardiac rehabilitation regimens also reduces morbidity, psychological distress, and some biological risk factors (Linden et al., 1996). For example, interventions combining psychosocial strategies such as stress management and behavioral risk factor reduction, including exercise, have been shown to reduce morbidity and favorably affect the index of myocardial ischemia in cardiac patients (Blumenthal et al., 1997). Despite such results, however, as few as 10 percent of all eligible patients who could potentially benefit from cardiac rehabilitation services actually participate in formal rehabilitation programs due to cost, inconvenience, or lack of motivation (Wenger et al., 1995). Such findings underscore the future importance of clinical management of disease that effectively integrates current medical regimens with knowledge of optimal motivational strategies for patients.

Family and Network Interventions

Chronically ill patients, especially with life-threatening diseases like cancer or AIDS, must contend with a series of stressful life events. Evidence suggests that availability of or increase in social support during times of stress may lessen or prevent mood disturbances, thereby improving chances of recovery and survival from cancer (Koopman et al., 1998). Overall social isolation is associated with a greater than twofold elevation in the relative risk of all-cause mortality, comparable to that associated with cigarette smoking or elevated serum cholesterol (House et al., 1988; see also Chapter 5). Although many studies suggest that the presence of social networks reduces mortality risk, most studies are limited by relying on one-time assessments of social support to predict disease outcome years later or use of inadequate proxy measures of social support (Spiegel and Kato, 1996). Studies are needed that systematically evaluate the benefits of intervening at the family or social network level. The studies of group support interventions suggest that such an approach would be worthwhile.

One program providing coping effectiveness training for men living with HIV includes an explicit social intervention component (Chesney et al., 1996). Individuals identify their support networks and characterize the persons in their networks into one of two groups of support providers: those who primarily provide problem-focused support, such as advice, and those who primarily provide emotion-focused support, such as listening and understanding. Although measures of the effectiveness of separate components in this program are not available, exit interviews with program participants indicate that they find the social intervention component to be especially helpful.

Families have been targeted in programs aimed at changing health risk behaviors of children. The involvement of at least one parent in programs addressing childhood obesity typically increases the effectiveness compared to controls where no parents are involved (Epstein et al., 1994). Evidence from one study comparing standard behavioral treatment with social support strategies suggests that involvement of friends as well as family members increases the effectiveness of intervention substantially (Wing and Jeffery, 1999). Of those recruited alone, 76 percent completed treatment and 24 percent maintained their weight loss in full from months 4 to 10, whereas of those recruited with friends 95 percent completed treatment and 66 percent maintained their full weight loss.

In general, however, families and proximal social networks, which are central to human health (see Chapter 5), have received comparatively little attention in the intervention realm. How spouses, parents, and children can contribute to each other's effective health practices (e.g., diet and exercise, adherence to treatment regimens, avoidance of harmful behaviors) is an important target for future inquiry.

Organization- and Population-Level Interventions

The classic examples of successful community interventions are the North Karelia Project (Pietinen et al., 1996; Puska and Koskella, 1985), the Stanford Three Community Study (Altman et al., 1987; Farquhar et al.,

1977), and the Stanford Five-City Project (Farquhar et al., 1990; see also Sorensen et al., 1998). All three targeted change and risk factors for coronary heart disease, including high blood pressure, elevated blood cholesterol levels, cigarette smoking, and obesity. The level of change observed in the North Karelia and Stanford Three Community Study, however, generally has not been replicated in subsequent community-based intervention trials. It should be noted that the level of motivation was high in North Karelia because of its identification as having the highest heart attack risk worldwide. Although community interventions have demonstrated that they can change health behaviors, the effectiveness and interactions among separate components of such programs are not well understood.

Work sites are now considered key channels for delivery of interventions designed to change behavior to prevent diseases and promote health among adult populations. Key targets for these workplace-based interventions include smoking cessation, improvement in diet, and physical activity (Sorensen et al., 1998). Other current lines of workplace research having potential to inform work site interventions are studies of stress and health risks in repetitive work and supervisory monitoring work (Lundberg and Johansson, 1999) as well as stress responses to low-status jobs and their links to musculoskeletal disorders (Lundberg, 1999). It is also important to note that, while programs in institutions have proven effective where studied as part of a specially funded effort, general adoption of successful programs into work site employee programs or school curricula has not frequently occurred.

Interventions can be classified according to increasing orders of coerciveness (e.g., degree to which they force behavior change). In the context of tobacco control the most coercive levels pertain to laws and regulations (Warner, 2000). These have contributed, along with other interventions, to considerable progress in tobacco control, with prevalence of smoking dropping from approximately 45 percent in 1963 (U.S. DHEW, 1964) to 25 percent in 1997 (CDC, 1999). With regard to early prevention, even modest increases in cigarette tax rates have been shown to reduce youth smoking (National Cancer Institute, 1993; Warner et al., 1995; Chaloupka and Warner, in press). Although the impact of rising prices is less evident for adults, smoking in adulthood is also responsive to price (Chaloupka and Warner, in press). The other principal regulatory intervention that affects smoking by adults is prohibition against smoking in public places. Ironically, indoor air laws were implemented for other reasons (i.e., to protect nonsmokers from the dangers of tobacco smoke), but they have along the way decreased smoking in the aggregate (Brownson et al., 1997) and for youth helped establish a nonsmoking social norm. These policy-level interventions warrant consideration in other public health problems, although lessons from tobacco control should proceed with caution (Warner, 2000).

KEY TRENDS

Largely due to the human genome project (Pennisi, 2000) and advances in diagnostic testing, it is increasingly possible to identify people's risk for certain diseases and conditions at earlier stages. For example, isolation of the BRCA1 gene, which affects susceptibility to breast and ovarian cancer, has led biotechnology companies to market genetic tests (see, e.g., Lerman et al., 1997). Early identification of vulnerability, however, can have mixed consequences. In addition to introducing the possibility of early treatment and possible cure, early diagnosis can discourage patients from seeking treatment. Cancer patients can face ostracism, dismissal, and hostility from others (Feldman, 1986), and awareness of this discrimination among patients living with chronic conditions such as HIV and cancer motivates many to choose not to disclose their status, even to health care providers (Chesney and Smith, 1999).

Past medical and psychosocial interventions have focused largely on the standard risk factors for chronic illness, such as inactivity, smoking, and unhealthy diet. These interventions, when studied and found to be effective, do not find their way into health plans for the individual. Psychosocial interventions for coping with chronic illnesses, such as cancer, or self-management of such chronic conditions as arthritis (Lorig et al., 1998) are also effective in improving functioning and quality of life; however, these also are not supported through health plans. There is a need to translate research into practice and to study the best mechanisms by which to achieve this objective.

This report highlights new social risk factors, including social isolation and lower socioeconomic status (SES). Apart from the group interventions for cancer or other conditions discussed earlier, little research has been conducted on social-level interventions. The effective strategies for building support systems or networks have not been identified. Nor have there been studies to evaluate interventions designed to address the risk associated with lower SES. As detailed in Chapter 8, racial/ethnic and SES variation is particularly salient in the context of smoking. For example, smoking prevalence is particularly high among Native Americans and Alaskans compared to other ethnic minorities (CDC, 1999). Since the anti-smoking campaign began in 1964, the change in smoking prevalence has also varied dramatically by educational level, falling nearly two-thirds among college graduates but only by one-sixth among those without a high school diploma (CDC, 1999). "In short, smoking has moved from an 'egalitarian' burden in the mid-1960s to a heavy weight today on those of low socioeconomic status" (Warner, 2000). This widening gap has received limited attention and clearly intersects with the problem of reducing social inequalities in health (see Chapter 7).

In addition to the needed emphasis on particular at-risk segments of society, there is also need for giving increased attention to interventions in families, organizations, and communities (see Sorensen et al., 1998). Given the growing awareness of the critical importance of social and contextual factors in health described in this report (see Chapters 3, 5, 6, and 7), consideration of a broader array of interventions is appropriate. The following elaborates this need.

Behavioral and psychosocial interventions historically were proposed as an alternative to biomedical approaches. Among the exceptions has been research on behavioral interventions to increase adherence to medical regimens. There is, however, a need to extend the work at the interface between behavioral and biomedical approaches. More sophisticated behavioral theories and strategies could, for example, be brought into play in studies of adherence, including the viewpoint that this is another health behavior that must be maintained over time. Similarly, biomedical approaches could be integrated with behavioral strategies to more effectively treat obesity, eating disorders, or cigarette smoking. Research investigating the efficacy of combined behavioral and pharmacological approaches often demonstrates a superiority for the combined approaches over either approach alone. Biobehavioral strategies could be extended to interventions directed at coping with chronic conditions and recovery from acute illness.

The behavioral interventions discussed in this chapter have been manual based but often delivered by professionals to individuals or groups, either separately or within work sites or schools. New technologies exist at various levels to offer innovative strategies at all levels. At the individual level, alpha-numeric pagers can prompt individuals to adhere to specific medication dosing schedules or to monitor blood glucose levels. Computers and telecommunications offer new opportunities for interactive decision making between patients and providers or for support among patient groups.

Similar programs need to be developed at the organizational and population levels. These programs would not need to treat all persons in the population the same way. Technology and self-selection would permit individuals or groups to obtain information tailored to their needs through community-level channels. Research indicates that such tailoring significantly improves the chances that recipients will thoughtfully consider the information and move toward self-assessment and intention to change (Kreuter et al., 1999).

People often have limited time, patience, and cognitive capacity for learning about health-related decisions. As a result, the content of health communications must be selected with great care. Risk, policy, and decision analysts have developed approaches to that selection process for communicating with professional audiences. These must be adapted to the needs of laypersons, recognizing the diversity of the personal circumstances, values, and knowledge levels that they may have (Fischhoff, 1999; Lipkus and Hollands, 1999; Schwartz et al., 1999; Vernon, 1999).

Collectively, these trends underscore the importance of the multilevel approach to health interventions. Here again the experience in smoking prevention and cessation is instructive. Extensive review of programs in this area (Warner, 2000) as well as their translation to clinical practice (U.S. Public Health Service Report, 2000) underscores the importance of grounding intervention programs in solid science and of approaching tobacco control via multipronged strategies (e.g., educational programs, media advertising, counseling, social support, pharmacotherapies for nicotine dependence, cigarette taxes, prohibition against smoking in public places). These various levels almost certainly reinforce each other, although further research is needed to evaluate the effectiveness of multiple intervention channels running simultaneously.

FUTURE RESEARCH NEEDS AND DIRECTIONS

Behavioral and social interventions have traditionally emphasized acute change. The implicit assumption has been that the individual, group, community, or population had some adverse approach to health that could be corrected with a brief program, often lasting 8 to 10 weeks. Thus, for example, the overweight people in the community would self-assess their eating habits and participate in that community program for a period of weeks, change their eating behavior, and sustain that change for life. Employees at the work site would start exercising and sustain that behavior. Patients coping with HIV/AIDS or cancer would learn new coping skills and apply them as their progressive illnesses presented new challenges over the years. There are some health behaviors that fit this acute intervention model better than others. Most health behaviors and certainly approaches to managing chronic conditions require a different model. There is an urgent need for new models of behavior change that address sustaining effort in the face of forever-changing personal, social, and environmental circumstances. The failure of our current models to address the dynamic of time and circumstance may explain why some models, such as the transtheoretical model of behavior change or "stages of change," while having considerable intuitive appeal, have proven not to be widely applicable. In recent years research on smoking (Herzog et al., 1999) and diet (Jeffery et al., 1999) found no association between stage and health outcomes achieved with intervention. (See, however, "Behavioral Factors" in Chapter 2 for more supportive evidence.)

In the early 1980s the National Heart, Lung, and Blood Institute and the National Cancer Institute suggested a sequence of research phases for development of programs effective in modifying behaviors (NHLBI, 1983). These phases range from hypothesis development (Phase I) and methods development (Phase II) through controlled intervention trials (Phase III) to studies in defined populations (Phase IV) and demonstration research (Phase V). The need to improve our understanding of mechanisms at the physiological, psychological, social, and population levels documented in this report, however, suggests that funding should be available for such integrative research. Pilot studies and small-group research must precede larger-scale studies. It is also important to note that some research problems and certain intervention approaches are optimally evaluated by randomized controlled clinical trials. Other problems and interventions, particularly those focusing at the organization or community level, may require new designs. Additional methods for demonstrating feasibility, sustainability, and cost effectiveness must be developed for population-level interventions.

There are four common features of population-level interventions that make traditional randomized control trials difficult, if not impossible:

1. The program contains multiple interventions acting simultaneously.
2. Participants are self-selected.
3. It is unknown whether the decision criteria used by volunteers are the same or different from those who do not participate.
4. A control group from the target population cannot be assembled.

Regarding the first feature, high-dimensional factorial experiments are required to assess the impact of each component intervention acting alone or in combination with other interventions. When the impact of a package of interventions is the primary concern, randomization in complex factorial designs is wasteful in time (taking many years to assess the effects of subsets of the full package) and resources.

With respect to the second feature, random assignment of persons to treatment and control groups can eliminate from consideration one or more central phenomena that require study. For example, in evaluating methadone maintenance programs, the target population is the set of chronic heroin users in a given community. Part of what one wants to understand is the characteristics of those who self-select to come into the program in the first place.

The third feature is related to the second in that it is useful to study the decision-making processes of volunteers versus nonvolunteers. Feature four is obviously outside the domain of a conventional randomized clinical trial. The investigator must make comparisons between the responses of voluntary participants and the known natural history of a given disease assessed in other studies.

Taken together, these attributes mean that multiple criteria should be used to evaluate the effectiveness of such interventions and that intervention outcomes should be compared with those of other programs or with outcomes absent of interventions (see Singer, 1986). Moreover, an administrative structure that is minimally intrusive to the patient may be of as much importance as the treatment itself. Randomized trials that included variations in administrative structure would be prohibitively costly. A more effective strategy is to combine performance-based ratings of program organization and implementation with outcome assessments (Singer, 1986). The complexity of such intervention programs suggests that what is deemed effective should be installed initially and that one or more components should be adjusted at regular intervals, based on outcome indices.

It should be recognized that intervention programs will seldom if ever be based on complete understanding of mechanisms at all levels described in this report. In this respect, intervention research is analogous to brain research, which often focuses on specific mechanisms in a particular group of cells or functional system without accounting for all interactions of that component with other parts of the brain or all processes within that component. Similarly, intervention research needs to selectively focus on specific mechanisms. Research designs should specify the mechanisms of interest and measures for assessing implementation of the designed intervention as well as health outcomes at appropriate levels.

The great successes of the past in convincing people to take better care of themselves have generally occurred when there was broad social consensus on appropriate behavior (even among those who were still acting otherwise). The persuasive approach, however, is less acceptable where such consensus is lacking. Individual circumstances may be sufficiently different that distinct courses of action may be indicated or there may be conflicting or culturally specific interpretations of the facts that might not be subject to reconsideration. The educational components of interventions must accommodate the full contextual setting. Overall, the need for longitudinal data, heterogeneous populations, and multiple intervention levels calls for integrative and linked studies to illuminate broad interventive targets, as described in this chapter. Development of an overall strategy and coordination of separate efforts will be of utmost importance. Across the entire spectrum of interventions, there is a great need to increase dissemination of preventive and treatment strategies that are found to be effective to the larger public.

RECOMMENDATIONS

The National Institutes of Health should support a new generation of intervention studies with the following emphases:

- development of strategies for extending successful social and behavioral interventions to more heterogeneous populations, including those focused on prevention via early identification of persons at risk: the design of interventions that take into account the dynamic and more chronic aspects of health should be given priority;
- expansion of implementation and dissemination activities so as to reduce the gap between research progress and practice;
- development of an overall strategy for intervention research that integrates behavioral, psychosocial, and biomedical approaches and spans multiple levels, from the individual to the societal;
- intervention research that capitalizes on new opportunities created by technological innovation should be given priority.

REFERENCES

Altman DG, Flora JA, Fortmann SP, Farguhar JW. 1987 "The cost-effectiveness of three smoking cessation programs" *American Journal of Public Health* 77/2:162-165.

Blumenthal JA, Jiang W, Babyak MA, Krantz DS, Frid DJ, Coleman RE, Waugh R, Hanson M, Appelbaum M, O'Connor C, Morris JJ. 1997 "Stress management and exercise training in cardiac patients with myocardial ischemia. Effects on prognosis and evaluation of mechanisms" *Archives of Internal Medicine* 157/19:2213-2223.

Brownson RC, Eriksen MP, David RM et al. 1997 "Environmental tobacco smoke: Health effects and policies to reduce exposures" *Annual Review of Public Health* 18:163-185.

Bruvold WH. 1993 "A meta-analysis of adolescent smoking prevention programs: A case study in Massachusetts" *American Journal of Public Health* 83/16:872-880.

CDC (Centers for Disease Control and Prevention). 1999 "Cigarette smoking among adults–United States, 1997" *Morbidity and Mortality Weekly Report* 48:993-996.

Chaloupka FJ, and Warner KE. In press "Economics of smoking" in Culyer AJ, Newhouse JP (eds.) *Handbook of Health Economics* (Amsterdam: Elsevier).

Chesney MA, Smith AW. 1999 "Critical delays in HIV testing and care: The potential role of stigma" *American Behavioral Scientist* 42/7:1162-1174.

Chesney MA, Folkman S, Chambers D. 1996 "Coping effectiveness training for men living with HIV: Preliminary findings" *International Journal of STD and AIDS* 7/suppl.2:75-82.

Chesney MA, Thurston RC, Thomas KA. 2001 "Creating social and public health environments to sustain behavior change: Lessons from obesity research" in Schneiderman N, Gentry J, da Silva JM, Speers M, Tomes H (eds.) *Integrating Behavioral and Social Sciences with Public Health* (Washington DC: American Psychological Association) pp. 31-50.

Compas BE, Haaga DA, Keefe FJ, Leitenberg H, Williams DA. 1998 "Sampling of empirically supported psychological treatments from health psychology: Smoking, chronic pain, cancer, and bulimia nervosa" *Journal of Consulting and Clinical Psychology* 66/1:89-112.

Craighead LW, Agras WS. 1991 "Mechanisms of action in cognitive-behavioral and pharmacological interventions for obesity and bulimia nervosa" *Journal of Consulting and Clinical Psychology* 59/1:115-125.

Epstein LH, Valoski A, Wing RR, McCurley J. 1994 "Ten-year outcomes of behavioral family-based treatment for childhood obesity" *Health Psychology* 13/5:373-383.

Farquhar JW, Fortman SP, Flora JA, Taylor CB, Haskell WL, Williams PT, Maccoby N, Wood PD. 1990 "Effects of community-wide education on cardiovascular disease risk factors: The Stanford Five-City Project." *Journal of the American Medical Association* 264/3:359-365.

Farquhar JW, Maccoby N, Wood PD, Alexander JK, Breitrose H, Brown BW Jr, Haskell WL, McAlister AL, Meyer AJ, Nash JD, Stern MP. 1977 "Community education for cardiovascular health" *Lancet* 1(8023):1192-1195.

Fawzy FI, Kemeny ME, Fawzy NW, Elashoff R, Morton D, Cousins N, Fahey JL. 1990 "A structured psychiatric intervention for cancer patients: II. Changes over time in immunological measures" *Archives of General Psychiatry* 47/8:729-735.

Feldman FL. 1986 "Female cancer patients and caregivers: Experiences in the workplace" *Women and Health* 11/3-4:137-153.

Fischhoff B. 1999 "Why (cancer) risk communication can be hard" *Journal of the National Cancer Institute Monographs* 25:1-7.

Gellert GA, Maxwell RM, Siegel BS. 1993 "Survival of breast cancer patients receiving adjunctive psychosocial support therapy: A 10-year follow-up study" *Journal of Clinical Oncology* 11/1:66-69.

Herzog TA, Abrams DB, Emmons KM, Linnan LA, Shadel WG. 1999 "Do processes of change predict smoking stage movements? A prospective analysis of the transtheoretical model" *Health Psychology* 18/4:369-375.

House JS, Landis KR, Umberson D. 1988 "Social relationships and health" *Science* 241/4865:540-545.

Jeffery RW, French SA, Rothman AJ. 1999 "Stage of change as a predictor of success in weight control in adult women" *Health Psychology* 18/5:543-546.

Kleinman A. 1981. *Patients and Healers in the Context of Culture* (Berkeley: University of California Press).

Kleinman A. 1989 *The Illness Narratives: Suffering, Healing, and the Human Condition* (New York: Basic Books).

Koopman C, Hermanson K, Diamond S, Angell S, Spiegel D. 1998 "Social support, life stress, pain and emotional adjustment to advanced breast cancer" *Psycho-Oncology* 7/2:101-111.

Kreuter MW, Bull FC, Clark EM, Oswald DL. 1999 "Understanding how people process health information: A comparison of tailored and nontailored weight-loss materials" *Health Psychology* 18/5:487-494.

Lerman C, Biesecker B, Benkendorf JL, Kerner J, Gomez-Caminero A, Hughes C, Reed MM. 1997 "Controlled trial of pretest education approaches to enhance informed decision-making for BRCA1 gene testing" *Journal of the National Cancer Institute* 89/2:148-157.

Linden W, Stossel C, Maurice J. 1996 "Psychosocial interventions for patients with coronary artery disease: A meta-analysis" *Archives of Internal Medicine* 156/7:745-752.

Lipkus IM, Hollands JG. 1999 "The visual communication of risk" *Journal of the National Cancer Institute Monographs* 25:149-162.

Lorig K, Gonzalez VM, Laurent DD, Morgan L, Loris BA. 1998 "Arthritis self-management program variations: Three studies. *Arthritis Care and Research* 11/6:448-454.

Lundberg U. 1999 "Stress responses in low-status jobs and their relationship to health risks: Musculoskeletal disorders. *Annals of the New York Academy of Sciences* 896:162-172.

Lundberg U, Johansson G. 1999 "Stress and health risks in repetitive work and supervisory monitoring work" in Backs RW and Boncsein W (eds.) *Engineering Psychophysiology: Issues and Applications* (Mahwah NJ: Lawrence Erlbaum) 339-359.

National Cancer Institute. 1993 *The Impact of Cigarette Excise Taxes on Smoking Among Children and Adults: A Summary Report of a National Cancer Institute Expert Panel* (Bethesda MD: Division of Cancer Prevention and Control, NCI).

Naughton J. 1992 "Exercise training for patients with coronary artery disease: Cardiac rehabilitation revisited" *Sports Medicine* 14/5:304-319.

NHLBI (National Heart, Lung, and Blood Institute). 1983 *Guidelines for Demonstration and Educational Research Grants* (Washington DC: U.S. Government Printing Office).

Pennisi E. 2000 "Human genome. Finally, the book of life and instructions for navigating it" *Science* 288/5475:2304-2307.

Puska P, Koskella K. 1985 "Community-based strategies to fight smoking: Experiences from the North Karelia Project in Finland" in A Blum (ed.) *The Cigarette Underworld* (Mahwah NJ: Lyle Stuart Inc.) pp.95-98.

Pietinen P, Vartiainen E, Seppanen R, Arro A, Puska P. 1996 "Changes in diet in Finland from 1972 to 1992: Impact on coronary heart disease risk" *Preventive Medicine* 25/3:243-250.

Schwartz L, Woloshin S, Welch G. 1999 "Risk communication in clinical practice" *Journal of the National Cancer Institute Monographs* 25:124-133.

Singer B. 1986 "Self-selection and performance-based ratings: A case study in program evaluation" in H Wainer (ed.) *Drawing Inferences from Self-Selected Samples* (New York: Springer-Verlag) pp.29-49.

Sorensen G, Emmons K, Hunt MK, Johnston D. 1998 "Implications of the results of community intervention trials" *Annual Review of Public Health* 19:379-416.

Spiegel D, Kato PM. 1996 "Psychosocial influences on cancer incidence and progression—Review" *Harvard Review of Psychiatry* 4/1:10-26.

Spiegel D, Bloom JR, Kraemer HC, Gottheil E. 1989 "Effect of psychosocial treatment on survival of patients with metastatic breast cancer" *Lancet* 2/8668:888-891.

Stevens VJ, Hollis JF. 1989 "Preventing smoking relapse, using an individually tailored skills-training technique" *Journal of Consulting and Clinical Psychology* 57/13:420-424.

U.S. DHEW (U.S. Department of Health, Education, and Welfare). 1964 *Smoking and Health: Report of the Advisory Committee to the Surgeon General of the Public Health Service* (Washington DC: U.S. Department of Health, Education, and Welfare, Public Health Service, Center for Disease Control) PHS Publication No. 1103.

U.S. DHHS (U.S. Department of Health and Human Services). 1994 *Preventing Tobacco Use Among Young People: A Report of the Surgeon General* (Washington DC: U.S. Government Printing Office, U.S. Department of Health and Human Services, Public Health Service, Centers for Disease Control, National Center for Chronic Disease Prevention and Health Promotion, Office of Smoking and Health).

U.S. DHHS (U.S. Department of Health and Human Services). 1996 *Smoking Cessation, Clinical Practice Guideline Number 18* Public Health Service, Agency for Health Care Policy and Research, Centers for Disease Control and Prevention. (Rockville MD: AHCPR Publication No. 96-0692).

U.S. Public Health Service Report. 2000 "A clinical practice guideline for treating tobacco use and dependence" *Journal of the American Medical Association* 283/24:3244-3254.

Velicer WF, Prochaska JO, Fava JL, Laforge RG, Rossi JS. 1999 "Interactive versus noninteractive interventions and dose-response relationships for stage-matched smoking cessation programs in a managed care setting" *Health Psychology* 18/1:21-28.

Vernon SW 1999 "Risk perception and risk communication for cancer screening behaviors: A review" *Journal of the National Cancer Institute Monographs* 25:101-118.

Warner KE. 2000 "The need for, and value of, a multi-level approach to disease prevention: The case of tobacco control" in Smedley BD and Syme SL (eds.) *Promoting Health: Intervention Strategies from Social and Behavioral Research* (Washington, DC: National Academy Press, Committee on Capitalizing on Social Science and Behavioral Research to Improve the Public's Health, Division of Health Promotion and Disease Prevention, Institute of Medicine) pp.326-352.

Warner KE, Chaloupka FJ, Cook PJ et al. 1995 "Criteria for determining an optimal cigarette tax: The economist's perspective" *Tobacco Control* 4:380-386.

Wenger NK, Forelicher ES, Smith LK, and the Cardiac Rehabilitation Guideline Panel of the Agency for Health Care Policy and Research. 1995 *Cardiac Rehabilitation* (Rockville MD: U.S. Department of Health and Human Services).

Wing RR, Jeffery RW. 1999 "Benefits of recruiting participants with friends and increasing social support for weight loss and maintenance" *Journal of Consulting and Clinical Psychology* 67/1:132-138.

10

Methodology Priorities

A central feature of each topic area in this report is a focus on complex dynamic systems. The conceptual formulation of such phenomena as predisease pathways, the influence of collective community properties on individual health, and resilience in the face of adversity involve integrating components of complex systems. Methodological innovation will be needed to achieve such integration. New measurement techniques and designs at both the animal and human levels are necessary to build bridges that link the social and psychological levels of description to biology. The specification of multiple methods to strengthen support for—or refutation of—proposed linkages among complex psychosocial and physiological systems (Kagan, 1999) is an important priority across the full range of phenomena discussed in this report. Finally, the objective of understanding complex systems at multiple levels of description poses new statistical challenges, beyond the reach of currently available techniques. These challenges extend to the need to design and evaluate multicomponent intervention studies.

We have intentionally refrained from putting forth a formal complex systems model incorporating the full range of phenomena discussed. This would be premature in topic areas that are in a state of flux, where new developments in the published literature appear weekly. The topics raised in this chapter are meant to be illustrative rather than comprehensive. The challenge of putting forth, analyzing, and defending (with empirical data) formal integrated systems models nonetheless represents an important priority in its own right.

CHARACTERIZING PATHWAYS

A variety of measurement and data analytic questions need to be resolved before multiple topics discussed in this report can be characterized with precision. Prediseases pathways, life histories of resilience in the face of adversity, and delineation of the biology of flourishing are among phenomena that call for methodological innovation. Priority topics include the need for greater investment in longitudinal designs, the measurement of numerous components of predisease pathways (e.g., childhood and early life influences, work and unemployment, positive health and resilience, collective properties and inequalities), the need to advance understanding of biological mechanisms, and the need for innovative methods of data analysis.

Investment in Longitudinal Studies

Implementation of the integrative perspective requires longitudinal assessment at multiple levels (psychosocial and biological) on the same individuals. This raises the practical question of how comprehensive such measurement can be on single populations and where inferences about pathways must be derived from studies of multiple populations. Concerning psychosocial and biological measures on the same population, several longitudinal studies illustrate needed future directions. The MacArthur Study of Successful Aging (Seeman et al., 1997) has measures of social integration and social support together with assays of glucocorticoids, catecholamines, cholesterol, glycosylated hemoglobin, blood pressure, and measures of adipose tissue deposition (thereby representing the preliminary operationalization of the concept of allostatic load) on the same individuals. A subsample of the Wisconsin Longitudinal Study (WLS) contains extensive psychosocial life history data (over a span of 40 years), community-level information, and multiple neurophysiological assessments (e.g., measures in the current allostatic load inventory, immune system assays of antibody responses to influenza and hepatitis A vaccine, EEG assessments of brain asymmetry, and fMRI assessments; e.g., Singer and Ryff, 1999). The 1999 round of the National Long Term Care Survey contains an extensive array of biomarkers, including assessment of apolipoprotein E (apoE) markers of genetic susceptibility to onset of Alzheimer's.[1] The Whitehall II study of British civil servants (Marmot et al., 1991) and the 1946 (Wadsworth and Kuh, 1997) and 1958 (Power and Matthews, 1998) British birth cohorts each have new biomarker data collections simultaneous

---

[1]The data are available electronically: Alzheimer's: http://cds.duke.edu/NLTCS-INTRO.HTML.

with the rich psychosocial and health measures that have been repeatedly collected in these studies. The ever more comprehensive biopsychosocial data available in the above studies provide far more informative under- standing of health pathways than can be obtained by creating synthetic cohorts by working across multiple studies.

The above examples, by no means exhaustive, clarify that extensive data collection is in fact feasible on factors that may initially appear to pose excessive respondent burden. A counterpoint to the above surveys (origi- nally oriented more toward psychosocial assessments), the Framingham Study (Dawber, 1980; Allaire et al., 1999) is rich in longitudinal health and biomarker assessments but weak in psychosocial information. Ideally, what is needed are both kinds of information assessed on the same individuals over time. Such data would greatly facilitate understanding the linkages between physiological, psychological, and sociological phenomena. Gene expression studies on large populations that, until a few years ago would not have been feasible, can also now be considered in future data collection, thanks to microarray chip technology (see Chapter 4). However, before delineating practical next steps regarding investment in longitudinal stud- ies, it would be useful to consider what an optimal portfolio of such studies might be.

First, it would be useful to have several birth cohorts specifically de- signed for the integrative agenda outlined in this report. This would in- clude DNA samples at birth with gene expression assessments over the life course. Measurement of successful functioning, or the lack thereof, of multiple physiological systems over the life course should be included. Collective properties of communities that influence these individuals (see Chapter 6) should be included together with a substantial array of psycho- logical and social assessments, as delineated in Chapters 2, 3, and 5. Some individuals in these birth cohorts would be exposed to "natural" experi- ments (e.g., legislation prohibiting smoking in public places, welfare re- form, regulation on the placement and protective features of toxic waste sites) having possible health consequences. Information about the impact of such policy-based, macro-level interventions on individuals should be assessed.

Second, beyond such comprehensive cross-time data collection, it would be desirable to have several explicit intervention studies in the portfolio, including some that are community based and involve multiple interven- tions acting simultaneously. The interventions should be of both the health- promoting and disease-preventing varieties (see Chapter 3). In addition, subsamples from such studies should be accessible for carrying out small- scale challenge studies, the purpose of which should be to link psychosocial challenges (e.g., marital conflict, performance evaluation) with biological antecedents and consequences. These purposive challenge studies should also be a part of protocols for the birth cohorts, where naturally occurring interventions predominate.

In-depth studies for some biomedical questions may not be practical within large longitudinal surveys or community-based intervention studies. Indeed, it is difficult to identify clear boundaries between the kinds of information usefully ascertained in large population studies and what must be left for investigations in smaller special populations. For this reason, we focus attention on the above broad categories of longitudinal studies as optimal targets and now turn to the practical processes of developing a useful portfolio.

To facilitate National Institutes of Health (NIH) engagement in support of future data collection for integrative studies, we recommend that a series of workshops be convened to identify the varieties of pathways (road maps) that are most in need of ongoing assessment. These workshops should also have the delineation of cost-effective optimal designs as a major objective. As indicated in other sections of this report (e.g., Chapters 2, 3, and 7), there are few extant longitudinal surveys (birth cohorts in particular) that could be the basis for implementing optimal designs. Thus, it would be important in such workshops to clarify the degree to which optimal designs could be achieved by piggybacking new measurements onto existing longitudinal studies. If resources were committed, for example, to separate surveys focused on children, midlife, and the elderly, which studies would represent the best opportunities for incorporating new instruments to build toward a picture of pathways? These workshops could also address what retrospective instruments (psychosocial and physiological signatures of past adversity and advantage) should be used in midlife and elderly population studies. The overall goal would be the specification of a long-term plan, with cost estimates, for implementing pathway studies. An important component of this recommendation would be the establishment of an ongoing advisory group that makes decisions adaptively, informed by accumulating evidence about the evolution of pathway studies. Measurement priorities related to components of pathways are identified below.

Measurement of Early Life and Childhood Influences

As documented in Chapter 2, prenatal experience plays a central role in interacting with the genome to influence brain development. These epigenetic influences in intrauterine life confer a set of predispositions that act across the life span to affect vulnerability for a host of chronic diseases. The quality of parenting behavior plays a central role in the development of stress regulatory systems. Children exposed to parenting characterized by conflict, aggression, and neglect showed disruption in the sympathetic adrenomedullary (SAM) and hypothalamic-pituitary-adrenal (HPA) regulatory systems. Conversely, positive maternal behavior protects against expression of genetic risk for serotonin dysregulation. Parenting also plays an important role in modifying genetically based temperamental differences in children. Such evidence indicates that empirical specification of pathways requires delineating best indicators of quality of parenting, temperaments, and family environments that can be utilized in large longitudinal studies. A companion set of physiological indicators of SAM and HPA system functioning is also required for use in large population studies. Protocols for salivary cortisol assessments, for example, on children are well developed (Gunnar, 1999). In addition, a broad array of biomarkers on children were collected as part of the NHANES III (U.S. DHHS, 1994).[2] What is required is the identification of subsets of biomarkers and protocols for their assessment that are most directly associated with psychosocial measures used to construct pathways.

Assessment of Personal Ties

Diverse forms of personal ties (e.g., mother-child attachment, spousal intimacy, close friendships, relationships with work colleagues) are central to pathway specifications relating to both negative and positive health outcomes (see Chapter 5). Recent literature suggests that the emotional aspects of personal ties are salient features linking the psychosocial level of description to biology and downstream health consequences (Ryff and Singer, in press). The study of emotion in personal ties requires further development at a conceptual and measurement level to relate emotions of both positive and negative valence to health. What is needed is a multi-method technology for assessing emotion in personal ties (e.g., survey instruments, focused interviews, writing tasks, experimental protocols) that together comprise comprehensive specification of pathways at the psychosocial level and their relationship to biology. A thorough investigation of the interplay between psychosocial assessments and neurophysiological measurements (e.g., left- versus right-side activation of the prefrontal cortex connected to the emotional aspects of personal ties; Ryff and Singer, in press) is an essential component of such a program of methodological development.

Assessment of Work and Unemployment Influences

There is an extensive literature associating adversity in the workplace and spells of unemployment with later-life chronic disease and mortality

---

[2]The data are available electronically: NHANES: www.cdc.gov/nchs/nhanes.htm.

(Marmot et al., 1997). In addition there are observational studies over short time intervals relating the pace and character of repetitive work tasks with mental health and musculoskeletal disorders (Lundberg, 1999). What is needed is delineation of the best measuring instruments for relating workplace and unemployment experience to the cumulative physiological risk (Grossi et al., 1998), such as allostatic level. This should include measures of cumulative adversity and responses to short-term challenges that are reflected in shifts in allostatic load over the life course.

Assessment of Positive Health and Resilience

Pathways of resilience and of persistent flourishing require specification of the principal positive features of lives at the individual and community levels that are most strongly associated with the maintenance of allostasis (see Chapter 3). Few extant studies discuss this kind of question. Nevertheless, the growing literature linking, for example, physical exercise and a variety of enriched environments with neurogenesis in animals suggests that this is the primary area for NIH-sponsored research. At the level of elderly human populations, the documentation of subgroups who maintain or improve their mental and/or physical health with increasing age (Ryff et al., 1998) also points to the need for expanded assessment of behavioral, psychological, social, and biological factors implicated in the maintenance of positive health. Delineation of the best measuring instruments at the psychosocial and biological levels to understand optimal biopsychosocial functioning in the face of adversity is a high priority for methodological development.

Particularly important is the need for research on the neurobiological mechanisms underlying the health benefits ensuing from behavioral and psychosocial influences. What are the actual processes (e.g., neural circuitry, endocrine and immune functions) through which behavioral (e.g., nutrition, exercise, stress management) and psychosocial (optimism, coping quality social ties) factors convey their health-promoting effects? This is a call to advance what is known about the physiological substrates of flourishing (Ickovics and Park, 1998; Ryff and Singer, 1998). Such inquiry has begun, as for example, in studies linking social supports to physiological processes (Seeman and McEwen, 1996; Uchino et al., 1996). These agendas have tended to focus, however, on the endocrinological and immunological correlates of relational conflict or caregiving demands (Kiecolt-Glaser et al., 1996, 1997), not relational strengths. Thus, there is a major need for new studies linking positive aspects of social relationships (attachment, affection, intimacy) to the mechanisms that underlie good health (Ryff and Singer, 2000). Animal research provides extremely valuable models for such explication of the mechanisms that connect positive social relations to health (Carter, 1998; Uvnas-Moberg, 1997, 1998).

Assessment of Collective Properties and Inequalities

Pathways specified by measures at the individual level must be linked to more macro-level phenomena that have been associated with individual-level health. Neighborhood-, city-, district-, county-, state-, and even national-level properties can have impact on the health status of entire communities as well as on the individual person. The existence of inequality reflects degrees of collective adversity relative to advantage and requires establishing profiles of individual histories that specify cross-domain influences. The growing body of instruments for measuring such phenomena as social cohesion and social control (Sampson et al., 1997) must be augmented with improved measures of community physical environments that bear directly on health risks (e.g., garbage in the streets; unsafe housing; accessibility of parks, recreational sites, and open spaces to more densely populated urban tracts; Institute of Medicine, 1999b).

The measurement of collective social characteristics themselves, including assessment of social well-being (Keyes, 1998), also needs refinement regarding their relationship to a diversity of health outcomes. Environments that are less divisive, less undermining of self-confidence, less conducive to antagonism, and more supportive of developing effective life skills are important goals for future research and intervention. Overall, the science of ecological assessment of social and physical environments (i.e., "ecometrics," see Chapter 6; Raudenbush and Sampson, 1999) relevant to health is underdeveloped and requires a concerted methodological effort bolstered by NIH support. Linking these collective measures to psychosocial and biological indicators at the individual level is a critical priority for characterizing the full range of pathways discussed in this report.

ADVANCING THE UNDERSTANDING OF BIOLOGICAL MECHANISMS

Going beyond statistical association to address the mechanisms by which behavioral, psychological, and social factors operate at various levels requires methodological development. In particular, ways of measuring the mechanisms that convey and moderate psychosocial influences on health are a top priority. The two most pressing needs are to understand the neural circuitry whereby environmental conditions and events affect emotions and downstream health outcomes, thereby extending the measurement of cumulative physiological burden and its consequences.

Neural Circuitry

Fundamental to developing pathway characterizations is an understanding of the chain of interrelationships from the macro-environmental level to the neural level. A central focus is on factors that influence psychological, social, and emotional processes, which when instantiated in the brain have downstream autonomic, endocrine, and immune consequences impinging on health. These psychosocial processes operate at an intermediate level that can be regarded as a necessary pathway through which external challenges influence health. In recent years there has been considerable progress in understanding the central neural circuitry that underlies emotion and affective style (Davidson, 1998). With this knowledge, it is possible to formulate mechanistic hypotheses about how life events and psychosocial factors, insofar as they influence brain circuitry, can have downstream effects on the periphery and thereby influence health.

Most extant research indicates variations in activation of the left prefrontal region with differences in approach-related positive affect (Sutton and Davidson, 1997). Decreased activation in this region is associated with increased vulnerability to depression, while increased activation is associated with dispositional positive affect and a coping style found to be protective against depressive symptomology (Tomarken and Davidson, 1994). Thus, given the same negative life events, an individual with baseline-left-anterior hypo-activation is hypothesized to show more intense depressive symptomology compared with a subject showing left-anterior hyper-activation.

From the perspective of brain function, resilience (see Chapter 3) may thus involve capacities to activate approach-related affective processes in the face of negative environmental stressors. Such capacities are likely products of enduring individual differences in dispositional mood and established patterns of emotional reactivity. Research has shown that subjects showing stable but extreme electrophysiological asymmetry differ in ratings of their own moods: those with extreme activation in the left prefrontal part of the brain showed both significantly more positive affect and significantly less negative affect than their right prefrontally activated counterparts (Tomarken et al., 1992).

To provide the necessary links between these aspects of affective neuroscience and pathway characterizations, it is essential to support the following research directions: (1) study profiles of brain circuitry over long time periods (prior work, described above, has focused on stability in asymmetries over relatively short intervals); (2) investigate whether greater left-sided prefrontal activation confers resilience in the face of cumulative negative life challenges; (3) map connections between hemispheric asymmetry and psychosocial variables (e.g., well-being, coping, quality of personal ties) and other biological indicators (allostatic load, measures of immune function). The development and implementation of protocols for longitudinal assessment on diverse populations (e.g., WLS, the 1946 and 1958 British birth cohorts) are a high priority. Resolution of these measurement issues would provide a critical link toward understanding the mechanisms by which proximate and distal social influences exert their health-transforming effects. An important advance would be instrumentation to facilitate EEG assessments on large populations under diverse environmental conditions. In particular, microminiaturization of the EEG recording and data storage units would make ambulatory measurement of brain activation in response to naturally occurring stimuli a reality.

Refinement in the Operationalization of Allostatic Load

Implicit in the concept of allostasis, "achieving stability through change" (see Chapter 3), are nature-nurture interactions in which genes are regulated by environmental factors, leading in the short run to adaptation and in the long run to increased risk for disease. A problem with the original conceptualization of allostatic load and its measurement, however, is that the components were not organized and categorized with regard to what each measure represents in the cascade of events that lead from allostasis to allostatic load. A step toward improving the formulation of culmulative physiological burden (McEwen and Seeman, 1999) has utilized the notion of primary mediators leading to primary effects and then to secondary outcomes, which lead finally to tertiary outcomes that represent actual diseases.

Primary mediators are chemical messengers released as part of allostasis. The present operationalization of allostatic load (Seeman et al., 1997, in press) has four such mediators: cortisol, epinephrine, norepinephrine, and DHEA-S. These mediators are accessible and relatively easy to collect and measure from body fluids, such as saliva, urine, and blood. Other mediators could include inflammatory cytokines and insulin-like growth factors. These and other future measures viewed as primary mediators have wide influences throughout the body and are useful in predicting a variety of secondary and tertiary outcomes.

Primary effects are cellular events, like enzymes, receptors, ion channels, or structural proteins induced genomically or phosphorylated via second messenger systems, that are regulated as part of allostasis by the primary mediators. These are not presently measured as part of an operationalization of allostatic load, although it may be desirable to include them in future formulations, as they are the basis for secondary and tertiary outcomes. Primary effects are organ and tissue specific, and as a result secondary and tertiary outcomes must be described at this level. The connections between primary effects and secondary and tertiary outcomes represent the current mechanistic research supported by NIH.

Secondary outcomes are integrated processes that reflect the cumulative outcome of the primary effects in a tissue/organ-specific manner in response to the primary mediators. Current operationalizations of allostatic load include the following secondary mediators, all of which are related to abnormal metabolism and risk for cardiovascular disease: waist/hip ratio, systolic and diastolic blood pressure, glycosylated hemoglobin, total/HDL cholesterol, and HDL cholesterol. In the future the secondary outcomes should be expanded in two directions. First, there is a need for more specific outcomes related to damage along the pathway of cardiovascular risk in relation to job stress and socioeconomic status (Markowe et al., 1985). Second, outcomes of cumulative burden in other systems, such as the brain and the immune system, are needed. For the brain, assessments of declarative and spatial memory have been employed to identify individual differences in brain aging, reflecting atrophy of the hippocampus and progressive elevation of cortisol (Lupien et al., 1998). For the immune system, integrated measures of the immune response such as delayed-type hypersensitivity (Dhabhar and McEwen, 1999) and immunization challenge (Dhabhar and McEwen, 1996) could reveal the impact of allostatic load on cellular and humoral immune function and help distinguish between the immuno-enhancing effects of acute stress and the immunosuppressive effects of chronic stress.

Tertiary outcomes are the actual diseases or disorders that are the result of the allostatic load predicted from the elevated/extreme values of the secondary outcomes and primary mediators. Thus far, the outcomes associated with high allostatic load have been cardiovascular disease, decreased physical capacity, severe cognitive decline, and mortality. Some redefinition of outcomes is needed. A stricter criterion based upon the definitions of primary, secondary, and tertiary outcomes would assign cognitive decline as a secondary outcome. Alzheimer's disease or vascular dementia would be included as tertiary outcomes, as these are cases where there is serious and permanent disease. Cancer would also be a tertiary outcome, clearly reflecting a compromised immune system as well as other systemic changes in endocrine and metabolic responses.

The above classification system should serve as a template for new studies relating progression from primary mediators to secondary outcomes and then to tertiary outcomes. New research should identify clusters of secondary outcomes that are relevant to particular diseases. Measurement of secondary outcomes at younger ages (as part of new operationalizations of allostatic load) must be implemented in longitudinal studies with tertiary outcomes at later ages. A more refined statistical methodology for combining information across primary mediators, primary effects, and secondary outcomes to establish a new index of allostatic load is a high priority for future research.

Beyond the above classification system and its attendant measurement problems are other methodological issues that warrant attention. First, the measures incorporated in the current operationalization of allostatic load are all based on resting level, or static, assessments. As a collectivity, they are supposed to represent the physiological signature of cumulative psychosocial adversity. This is only one aspect of allostatic load (McEwen and Seeman, 1999). Equally important is abnormal transient response of primary mediators to specific challenges because the repeated overactivity of a physiological system is a source of allostatic load (McEwen, 1998). Impaired transient response to acute challenge should be part of the physiological signature of cumulative adversity. Protocols in animals and humans are needed to document the phenomena and lead to an index of allostatic load incorporating both resting level and transient response measures.

A second missing feature of current operationalization of allostatic load is the specification and implementation of a defensible set of indicators for children. The extant indicators were developed for and calibrated on a longitudinal study of the elderly (Seeman et al., 1997). The same indicators have been used on a midlife sample (ages 59-60; Singer and Ryff, 1999), and a slightly modified operationalization has been utilized in the Normative Aging Study (Kubzansky et al., 1999). A comparison of the distribution of responses across these samples suggests that an age-specific specification of allostatic load would be appropriate. Since a characterization must involve physiological processes that evolve over the life course, the development of a whole-life animal model of allostatic load is likely to yield major payoff in developing the human analog. This would entail setting up experimental protocols that vary the frequency and types of psychosocial challenges to which the animals are exposed over their lives. It would also require age-dependent specification of the various components of the classification system described above.

A third aspect of the further operationalization of allostatic load that warrants further investigation is gender differences in resting levels and in transient response to challenges of particular primary mediators and secondary outcomes. For example, a higher proportion of elderly women show elevated levels of cortisol, epinephrine, and norepinephrine and low levels of DHEA-S. Elderly men tend to have elevated levels of syndrome X markers with greater frequency than women. In response to a 30-minute cognitive challenge, younger men showed greater cortisol reactivity than women. However, in elderly populations the pattern is reversed, with elderly women showing greater transient responses (Seeman et al., in press.)

There is a pressing need to specify protocols that would clarify the scope and character of age-specific gender differences in the components of a more refined specification of allostatic load.

The fourth challenge is the integration of knowledge about environmental influences on primary, secondary, and tertiary outcomes with the wealth of information coming from the human genome project. The ultimate goal of mapping the human genome is to enable medical science to unravel the genes that are involved in disease processes as well as the genes that help protect the body from disease. Such genes may be involved at any or all stages of the life course. Regulation of these genes is one of the greatest challenges facing biomedical science in this century.

A few words are in order about statistical analyses pertaining to the current formulation of allostatic load and its further development and operationalization. The primary and secondary mediators linked to secondary and tertiary outcomes represent a system of multiple indicators reaching high risk levels over time and subsequently influencing diverse kinds of outcomes. Organizing these dynamics in a comprehensive statistical framework could involve the use of structural equation modeling, including the incorporation of latent variables to represent unmeasured biological parameters. Development and implementation of such a framework are important aspects of operationalizing the notion of cumulative physiological risk, for which allostatic load is an illustrative beginning.

METHODS OF DATA ANALYSIS

The statistical challenges associated with pathway characterizations center around the necessity of developing new person-centered methods for representing the complex multidimensional and multilevel dynamics described throughout this report. Priorities in this area focus on three interrelated topics. First is the need to further develop both agglomerative and partition-based strategies for specifying categories of pathways. Second, new modeling, estimation, and testing protocols are required to carry out multilevel analyses that incorporate many of the nonlinearities within and between collective and individual-level descriptions of pathway components. Third, we require effective strategies for integrating numerical and narrative information as part of pathway characterizations. This integration includes the use of narratives in two forms: the construction of narratives by an investigator as part of a data analytic strategy and the analysis of narratives as data. These priorities are described in detail in the following three subsections.

Categories of Pathways

For an individual, a pathway specification at the psychosocial level consists of a chronology of the person's experience (where adversity and advantage interdigitate and sometimes run in parallel) across multiple life domains. There are feedback effects in which deteriorating health influences the extent and nature of subsequent adversity, and sustained positive experience can promote improvements in health. Similarly chronic adversity can promote deterioration in health, while high levels of mental and physical health can facilitate advantageous experience. The details of these individual histories are highly idiosyncratic. Thus, in specifying pathways to given health outcomes, strategies are required for abstracting and aggregating multiple histories so that empirically defined categories of histories emerge, in each of which individuals are regarded as approximate matches to one another. Statistical methodologies for the formation of coherent categories of pathways based on complex life histories are in their infancy. Such strategies are broadly referred to as person-centered methods, and they differ in both detail and objective from the widely available variable-centered techniques (Abbott and Hrycak, 1990; Cairns et al., 1998; Giele and Elder, 1998; Singer et al., 1998). The extant corpus of methods represents two distinct perspectives with the same basic objective. One set of methods starts with fine-grained individual case histories and aggregates up to categories of pathways. These are exemplified by the optimal matching (Abbott and Hrycak, 1990; Abbott and Barman, 1997), event-structure analysis (Griffin, 1993), and hybrid narrative/number-analytic techniques (Singer et al., 1998). The full individual history is the basic unit of analysis for all these methods. In optimal matching, for example, a metric is imposed on the set of possible histories. Those histories that fall within a prescribed small distance of one another are then identified as members of a common equivalence class (i.e., small idiosyncratic details that differ from one history to the next are disregarded and a more aggregate set of patterns is identified). There is an inevitable tension between the desire to preserve the nuances of an individual history and the necessity of disregarding some if aggregate categories are to be generated. The choice of metric reflects the features of histories to be emphasized in an aggregate category.

A second set of methods partitions the space of individual histories into successively more homogeneous categories, the final product being the desired pathway representations (Breiman et al., 1984; Zhang and Singer, 1999; Manton et al., 1994). Both of these classes of person-centered methods are substantially underdeveloped relative to the complexity of histories that would be the raw ingredients for longitudinal data analysis as outlined above. Furthermore, there are virtually no studies comparing and contrasting the scope and limitations of each perspective when applied to the same data set. Advancing person-centered statistical methodologies is essential for carrying out the empirical programs that appear throughout this report.

Nonlinearities

There is a growing set of applications of multilevel linear statistical models to quantify the impact of community-level indicators on individual experience and health (Malmstrom et al., 1999; Sampson et al., 1997; Yen and Kaplan, 1999). Several investigators (Manton et al., 1994; Breiman et al., 1984; Zhang and Singer, 1999) have called attention to the fact that the effect of substantial nonlinearities in the actual phenomena could be masked by the use of such over simplified models. Thus, it is imperative to expand the person-centered methodologies to incorporate collective properties of communities as they impact on individual-level experience. The multiple measurement strategies in the work on "ecometrics" as recently put forth by Raudenbush and Sampson (1999; see Chapter 6) must be linked systematically to the individual-level pathway construction methods. Another possible resource is the growing methodology of integrated assessment, drawing upon Bayesian approaches (e.g., influence diagrams) to combine research results from diverse disciplines (e.g., Clemen, 1991; Dowlatabadi and Morgan, in press; Howard, 1989). Applied most widely to complex environmental problems, with their nonlinearities, integrated assessments are increasingly being conducted for social-psychological domains, and their interaction with natural systems (e.g., Casman et al., 2000; Fischhoff, 2000; Fischhoff et al., 1998).

Person-Centered Narratives

Some of the extant person-centered methods use narrative information in two ways: (1) narratives based on interviews comprise part of the raw data that are to be combined with quantitative information in the process of pathway construction and (2) narratives describing whole lives, or major segments of them, are constructed by the analyst from long sequences of numerical information representing the longitudinal survey responses of a single individual. Under the latter the construction of narratives is part of an analytical strategy designed to formulate a coherent picture of a life history as it relates to physiology and health outcomes. Effectively integrating narratives as data, narratives constructed as part of an analytical strategy, and numerical information is a major challenge in pathway specification urgently in need of research support. Some movement in this direction is already apparent from recent (1999) planning workshops convened by the National Institute of Mental Health, but the general area is largely uncharted and is in need of much broader support.

DESIGN AND EVALUATION OF INTERVENTION PROGRAMS

Many of the most effective health promotion and disease prevention programs in the past have involved the use of multiple interventions acting simultaneously and/or in sequence (Watson, 1953; Warner, 2000). Voluntary self-selection into the programs is frequently a criterion for participation, thereby making controlled randomized trials impossible as a strategy for evaluation. Rehabilitation programs for chronic alcoholics, methadone maintenance programs for rehabilitation of heroin addicts, and family planning programs are among the many examples of interventions of this character (Singer, 1986). Self-selection is viewed in many quarters (Lipsey and Cordray, 2000) as a source of bias in assessing the impact of interventions. For programs of the type mentioned above, voluntary self-selection is part of the overall process to be studied. What is needed are defensible strategies for designing and evaluating complex intervention programs where self-selection is a criterion for entry into the program. A quite sophisticated labor economics literature on this topic has developed in the context of evaluating manpower training programs (Heckman and Smith, 1995). There is very little of similar character focused on health-based interventions where the details and level of complexity differ substantially from the labor economics context. Among the many issues that require attention is determining when one can defensibly ascertain the relative impact of a given intervention that is part of a package of interventions. A second important issue is that many successful multicomponent interventions in the past involved adaptive designs where the interventions were tuned experimentally, often over periods of several years, before optimal responses were obtained (Watson, 1921, 1953). In an environment where funding is linked to having all of the intervention structure specified a priori, packages of interventions that might be effectively tuned to optimal settings on given populations are seriously undermined. To broaden the base of design and analysis of multiple-component intervention programs, a series of methodological workshops should be convened to delineate funding priorities that would advance this subject on a broad scale. Many of the intervention programs implied by the discussion throughout this report are of the primary prevention variety. The methodology for effective evaluation of such programs is very underdeveloped and represents a pressing need.

Complementary to the need for population-level program evaluation strategies is the need to advance methodology focused on the information required by clinicians to guide patient management. Controlled randomized trials of pharmacological therapies usually focus on evaluating efficacy of a single drug as it performs "on average" in a population vastly more heterogeneous than the single patient of interest to the clinician. The standard clinical question is to ascertain how the contemplated therapy performed on a population of approximate matches, in terms of clinically relevant history, to a given patient (Horwitz et al., 1996, 1997, 1998). A single pharmacological agent is rarely the only intervention at issue. What the physician—and patient—need to know is how various packages of co-therapies perform on approximate matches to the given patient for whom an intervention program is being contemplated. Strategies for the assessment of packages of co-therapies that are tuned to the information needs of clinicians are in serious need of development. They represent the clinical counterpart to the evaluation methodology for multicomponent primary prevention programs described above. Serious attention should be given to this much neglected but ever more important aspect of providing effective curative medicine for the U.S. population.

Various NIH institutes support research designed to improve health-related decision making. We support the priority that NIH has set on developing better ways of presenting health care communications to lay people, especially the presentation of unfamiliar outcomes, processes, and units or comparisons (Fischhoff, 1999; Marcus, 1999; Woloshin and Schwartz, 1999). Attention also needs to be given to appropriate strategies in situation where causes, mechanisms, and outcomes are not viewed with broad consensus. In such situations the success of interventions cannot be evaluated simply in terms of how many individuals followed a common path. Rather, we need ways to evaluate our success in helping people to reach personally appropriate health decisions, ones that they understand, can live with, and are able to implement (e.g., Croyle and Lerman, 1999; Fischhoff, 1992; Rimer, 1995). Although health communications can be viewed in purely cognitive terms, they also touch the full human experience: not just the development of competency but the relationship between intellectual competence and self-efficacy needed for action, affective responses, and their impact on well-being (e.g., Baum et al., 1997; Institute of Medicine, 1999a). We recommend that research on these issues be encouraged and expanded.

RECOMMENDATIONS

New measurement techniques and designs for both animal and human studies are necessary to build bridges that will link behavioral, psychological, and social levels of analysis to multiple levels of biology (organ systems, cellular, molecular). This broad purview underscores the need for methodologies that are responsive to the functioning of complex dynamic systems through time. The emphasis on pathways in this report also implies a need for statistical methodologies that can specify pathway trajectories, address nonlinearities in diverse indicators, and incorporate narratives as sources of data. NIH should support methodological initiatives in three broad areas:

1. refined operationalization of allostatic load that takes explicit account of the cascade of events from allostasis to cumulating load; ambulatory assessments and responses to transient challenges should be given consideration as potential components of improved measures of allostatic load.

2. development of person-centered statistical methodologies to facilitate characterizations of predisease and positive health pathways that link behavioral, psychosocial, environmental, and biological levels of analysis;

3. development of design, implementation, and analysis strategies for multiple-component interventions where, to obtain optimal outcomes, allowance is made for adaptive, dynamic tuning of the interventions.

REFERENCES

Abbott A, Barman E. 1997 "Sequence comparison via alignment and Gibbs sampling: A formal analysis of the emergence of the modern sociological article" in Raftery A (ed.).*Sociological Methodology* (Washington DC: American Sociological Association) 47-87.

Abbott A, Hrycak A. 1990 "Measuring resemblance in sequence data: An optimal matching analysis of musicians' careers" *American Journal of Sociology* 96:144-185.

Allaire SH, LaValley MP, Evans SR, O'Connor GT, Kelly-Hayes M, Meenan RF, Levy D, Felson DT. 1999 "Evidence for decline in disability and improved health among persons aged 55 to 70 years: The Framingham Heart Study" *American Journal of Public Health* 89/11:1678-1683.

Baum A, Friedman AL, Zakowski SG. 1997 "Stress and genetic testing for disease risk" *Health Psychology* 16/1:8-19.

Breiman L, Friedman J, Olshen R, Stone C. 1984 *Classification and Regression Trees* (Belmont CA: Wadsworth Publishing Co.).

Carter CS. 1998 "Neuroendocrine perspectives on social attachment and love" *Psychoneuroendocrinology* 23/8:779-818.

Cairns R, Xie H, Leung MC. 1998 "The popularity of friendship and the neglect of social networks: Toward a new balance" *New Directions for Child Development* Summer/ 80:25-53.

Casman E, Fischhoff B, Palmgren C, Small M, Wu F. 2000 "Integrated risk model of a drinking waterborne cryptosporidiosis outbreak" *Risk Analysis* 20:493-509.

Clemen RT. 1991 *Making Hard Decisions: An Introduction to Decision Analysis* (Boston: PWS-Kent Publishing Co.).

Croyle RT, Lerman C. 1999 "Risk communication in genetic testing for cancer susceptibility" *Journal of the National Cancer Institute Monographs* 25:59-66.

Dawber T. 1980 *The Framingham Study* (New York: Oxford University Press).

Davidson, RJ. 1998 "Affective style and affective disorders: Perspectives from affective neuroscience" *Cognition and Emotion* 12:307-330.

Dhabhar F, McEwen BS. 1996 "Moderate stress enhances and chronic stress suppresses, cell-mediated immunity in vivo" *Society of Neuroscience* 22/536.5:1350.

Dhabhar F, McEwen BS. 1999 "Enhancing versus suppressive effects of stress hormones on skin immune function" *Proceedings of the National Academy of Sciences of the United States of America* 96:1059-1064.

Dowlatabadi H, Morgan MG. In press *Integrated Assessment* (New York: Cambridge University Press).

Fischhoff B. 1992 "Giving advice: Decision theory perspectives on sexual assault" *American Psychologist*.47/4:577-588.

Fischhoff B. 1999 "Why (cancer) risk communication can be hard" *Journal of the National Cancer Institute Monographs* 25:7-13.

Fischhoff B. 2000 "Scientific management of science?" *Policy Sciences* 33:73-87.

Fischhoff B, Downs JS, Bruine-de-Bruin W. 1998 "Adolescent vulnerability: A framework for behavioral interventions" *Applied and Preventive Psychology* 7/2:77-94.

Giele J, Elder G. 1998 *Methods of Life Course Research: Qualitative and Quantitative Approaches* (Thousand Oaks CA: Sage Publications).

Griffin L. 1993 "Narrative, event structure analysis, and causal interpretation in historical sociology" *American Journal of Sociology* 98:1094-1133.

Grossi A, Ahs A, Lundberg U. 1998 "Psychological correlates of salivary cortisol excretion among unemployed men and women" *Integrative Physiological and Behavioral Science* 33:249-263.

Gunnar M. 1999 "Early adversity and the development of stress reactivity and regulation" in Nelson CA (ed.) *The Effects of Adversity on Neurobehavioral Development: Minnesota Symposia on Child Psychology,* vol. 31 (Mahwah NJ: Lawrence Erlbaum).

Heckman J, Smith JA. 1995 "Assessing the case for social experiments" *Journal of Economic Perspectives* 9/2:85-110.

Horwitz RI, Singer BH, Makuch RW, Viscoli CM. 1996 "Can treatment that is helpful on average be harmful to some patients? A study of the conflicting information needs of clinical inquiry and drug regulation" *Journal of Clinical Epidemiology* 49/4:395-400.

Horwitz RI, Singer BH, Makuch RW, Viscoli CW. 1997 "On reaching the tunnel at the end of the light" *Journal of Clinical Epidemiology* 50/5:753-755.

Horwitz RI, Singer BH, Makuch RW, Viscoli CM. 1998 "Clinical versus statistical considerations in the design and analysis of clinical research" *Journal of Clinical Epidemiology* 51/4:305-307.

Howard RA. 1989 "Knowledge maps" *Management Science* 35:903-922.

Ickovics JR, Park CL. 1998 "Paradigm shift: Why a focus on health is important" *Journal of Social Issues* 54:237-244.

Institute of Medicine. 1999a *Adolescent Decision Making* (Washington DC: National Academy Press).

Institute of Medicine. 1999b *Toward Environmental Justice* (Washington DC: National Academy Press).

Kagan J. 1999 *Three Seductive Ideas* (Cambridge MA: Harvard University Press).

Keyes CLM. 1998 "Social well-being" *Social Psychology Quarterly* 61:121-140.

Kiecolt-Glaser JK, Glaser R, Gravenstein S, Malarkey WB, Sheridan J. 1996 "Chronic stress alters the immune response to influenza virus vaccine in older adults." *Proceedings of the National Academy of Sciences of the United States of America* 93:3043-3047.

Kiecolt-Glaser JK, Glaser R, Cacioppo JT, MacCallum RC, Snydersmith M, Cheongtag K, Malarkey WB. 1997 "Marital conflict in older adults: Endocrinological and immunological correlates" *Psychosomatic Medicine* 59:339-349.

Kubzansky L, Kawachi I, Sparrow D. 1999 "Socioeconomic status and risk factor clustering in the Normative Aging Study: Any help from the concept of allostatic load?" *Annals of Behavioral Medicine* 21/4:330-338.

Lipsey MW, Cordray DS. 2000 "Evaluation methods for social intervention" *Annual Review of Psychology* 51:345-375.

Lundberg U. 1999 "Stress responses in low-status jobs and their relationship to health risks: Musculoskeletal disorders" *Annals of the New York Academy of Sciences* 896:162-172.

Lupien SJ, DeLeon MJ, De Santi S, Convit A, Tarshish C, Nair NPV, Thakur M, McEwen BS, Hauger RL, Meaney MJ. 1998 "Cortisol levels during human aging predict hippocampal atrophy and memory deficits" *Nature Neuroscience* 1:69-73.

Malmstrom M, Sundquist J, Johansson SE. 1999 "Neighborhood environment and self-reported health status: A multi-level analysis" *American Journal of Public Health* 89/8:1181-1186.

Manton KG, Woodbury M, Tolley D. 1994 *Statistical Applications Using Fuzzy Sets* (New York: John Wiley and Sons).

Markowe HLJ, Marmot MG, Shipley MJ, Bulpitt CJ, Meade TW, Stirling Y, Vickers MV, Sernmence A. 1985 "Fibrinogen: A possible link between social class and coronary heart disease" *British Medical Journal* 291:1312-1314.

Marcus AC. 1999 "New directions for risk communication research" *Journal of the National Cancer Institute Monographs* 25:35-42.

Marmot MG, Smith GD, Stansfield S, Patel C, North F, Head J, White I, Brunner E, Feeney A. 1991 "Health inequalities among British civil servants: The Whitehall II study" *Lancet* 337/8754:1387-1393.

Marmot MG, Bosma H, Hemingway H, Brunner E, Stansfield S. 1997 "Contribution of job control and other risk factors to social variations in coronary heart disease incidence" *Lancet* 350:235-239.

McEwen BS. 1998 "Protective and damaging effects of stress mediators" *New England Journal of Medicine* 338/3:171-179.

McEwen BS, Seeman T. 1999 "Protective and damaging effects of mediators of stress: Elaborating and testing the concepts of allostasis and allostatic load" *Annals of New York Academy of Sciences* 896:30-47.

Power C, Matthews S. 1998 "Accumulation of health risks across social groups in a national longitudinal study" in Strickland SS, Shetty PS (eds.). *Human Biology and Social Inequality* (Cambridge U.K.: Cambridge University Press) 33-56.

Raudenbush SW, Sampson RJ. 1999 "Ecometrics: Toward a science of assessing ecological settings, with application to the systematic social observation of neighborhoods" *Sociological Methodology* 29:1-41.

Rimer BK. 1995 "Putting the 'informed' in informed consent about mammography" *Journal of the National Cancer Institute* 87/10:703-704.

Ryff CD, Singer BH. 1998 "The contours of positive human health" *Psychological Inquiry* 9:1-28.

Ryff CD, Singer BH. 2000 "Interpersonal flourishing: A positive health agenda for the new millennium" *Personality and Social Psychology Review* 4:30-44.

Ryff CD, Singer BH. In press "The role of emotion on pathways to positive health" in Davidson RJ, Goldsmith HH, Scherer K (eds.). *Handbook of Affective Science* (New York: Oxford University Press).

Ryff CD, Singer BH, Love GD, Essex MJ. 1998 "Resilience in adulthood and later life: Defining features and dynamic processes" in Lomranz J (ed.). *Handbook of Aging and Mental Health: An Integrative Approach* (New York: Plenum) 69-96.

Sampson RJ, Raudenbush, JD, Earls F. 1997 "Neighborhoods and violent crime: A multi-level study of collective efficacy" *Science* 227/5328:918-924.

Sampson RJ, Morenoff JD, Earls F. 1999 "Beyond social capital: Spatial dynamics of collective efficacy for children" *American Sociological Review* 64:633-660.

Seeman TE, McEwen BS. 1996 "Impact of social environment characteristics on neuroendocrine regulation" *Psychosomatic Medicine* 58:459-471.

Seeman TE, Singer BH, Rowe JW, Horwitz RI, McEwen BS. 1997 "The price of adaptation—allostatic load and its health consequences" *Archives of Internal Medicine* 157:2259-2268.

Seeman TE, Singer BH, Wilkinson RW, McEwen BS. In press "Gender differences in age-related changes in HPA axis reactivity" *Psychoneuroendocrinology.*

Singer B. 1986 "Self-selection and performance-based ratings: A case study in program evaluation" in Wainer H (ed.). *Drawing Inferences from Self-Selected Samples* (New York: Springer-Verlag) 29-49.

Singer B, Ryff CD. 1999 "Hierarchies of life histories and associated health risks" *Annals of the New York Academy of Sciences* 896:96-115.

Singer B, Ryff CD, Carr D, Magee W. 1998 "Linking life histories and mental health: A person-centered strategy" in Raftery A (ed.). *Sociological Methodology* (Washington DC: American Sociological Association) 1-51.

Sutton SK, Davidson RJ. 1997 "A biological substrate of the behavioral approach and inhibitor systems" *Psychological Science* 8:204-210.

Tomarken AJ, Davidson RJ. 1994 "Frontal brain activation in repressors" *Journal of Abnormal Psychology* 103:339-349.

Tomarken AJ, Davidson RJ, Wheeler RE, Doss RC. 1992 "Individual differences in anterior brain asymmetry and fundamental dimensions of emotion" *Journal of Personality and Social Psychology* 76:830-838.

Uchino BN, Cacioppo JT, Kiecolt-Glaser JK. 1996 "The relationship between social support and physiological processes: A review with emphasis on underlying mechanisms and implications for health" *Psychological Bulletin* 119:488-531.

U.S. DHHS (U.S. Department of Health and Human Services). 1994 *Vital and Health Statistics: Plan and Operation of the Third National Health and Nutrition Examination Survey, 1988-1994* (Washington DC: U.S. Department of Health and Human Services).

Uvnas-Moberg K. 1997. "Physiological and endocrine effects of social contact" *Annals of the New York Academy of Sciences* 807:146-163.

Uvnas-Moberg K. 1998 "Oxytocin may mediate the benefits of positive social interaction and emotions." *Psychoneuroendocrinology* 23:819-835.

Wadsworth MEJ, Kuh DJL. 1997 "Childhood influences on adult health: A review of recent work from the 1946 National Birth Cohort Study, the MRC national survey of health and development" *Pediatric Perinatal Epidemiology* 11:2-20.

Warner KE. 2000 "The need for, and value of a multi-level approach to disease prevention: The case of tobacco control" in Smedley BD and Syme SL (eds.). *Promoting Health: Intervention Strategies from Social and Behavioral Research* (Washington DC: National Academy Press) 326-352.

Watson, M. 1921 *The Prevention and Control of Malaria in the Federated Malay States: A Record of Twenty Years of Progress* (London: John Murray).

Watson M. 1953 *African Highway: The Battle for Health in Central Africa* (London: John Murray).

Woloshin S, Schwartz LM. 1999 "How can we help people make sense of medical data?" *Effective Clinical Practice* 2/4:176-83.

Yen IH, Kaplan GA. 1999 "Neighborhood social environment and risk of death: Multilevel evidence from the Alameda County study" *American Journal of Epidemiology* 149/10:898-907.

Zhang H, Singer B. 1999 *Recursive Partitioning in the Health Sciences* (New York: Springer-Verlag).

11

Research Infrastructure

S everal fundamental elements are needed to carry out the thematic priorities of this report. These include maintaining suitable study populations for long-term multilevel human and animal research, marshalling underutilized sources of clinical data, collecting new data on community-based interventions, and fostering scientists capable of working across multiple levels of analysis in the social, behavioral, and biomedical sciences.

HIGH-PRIORITY HUMAN AND ANIMAL POPULATIONS

It is essential to develop a mechanism for sustained core support of human and animal study populations, data bases, and laboratory animal colonies that can be used to study the integrated biopsychosocial pathways to diverse outcomes of both positive and negative valence.

The relevant human populations are of two interrelated kinds: (1) longitudinal surveys, preferably involving multiple birth cohorts, based on sampling from population registries at the individual level; and (2) community samples, such as the Chicago Neighborhood Project (Sampson et al., 1997), the Los Angeles Family and Neighborhood Study, and the Framingham Study (Dawber, 1980).[1] Community-level samples facilitate

---

[1]The data are available electronically: Los Angeles Family and Neighborhood Study: http://www.rand.org/lafans.html; Framingham Study: http://www.framingham.com/heart/.

the study of collective properties of populations and local physical surroundings as they influence individual and overall population-level health. At least two options are available for developing core samples to facilitate the kinds of studies prioritized in this report. One option is to start new birth cohorts and community studies that are responsive to the integrated biopsychosocial lines of inquiry. The second is to take existing longitudinal and community studies that have strengths in particular areas (e.g., psychosocial factors) and add biomedical factors to them. In the case of the Framingham Study, for example, psychosocial data would be needed to augment the superb biomedical assessments that have been the basis for this study from its inception.

As indicated in Chapters 2 and 3, there are few extant longitudinal samples that could be, even in principle, the basis for empirical characterizations of pathways over major portions of people's lives. The 1946 and 1958 British birth cohorts (Power and Matthews, 1998; Wadsworth and Kuh, 1997), the Wisconsin Longitudinal Survey (WLS; Hauser et al., 1993), the Alameda County Study (Berkman and Breslow, 1983), the Baltimore Longitudinal Study of Aging (National Institute on Aging, 1991), and the Harvard Mastery of Stress Study (Russek and Schwarz, 1997) are prominent examples of long-term studies that could be included in the core investigations of biopsychosocial pathways. Furthermore, it would be useful to add biomarker and other health-related data to the National Longitudinal Survey (NLS), the Panel Study of Income Dynamics (PSID), the Health and Retirement Survey (HRS), the National Survey of Families and Households (NSFH), and the Survey of Income and Program Participation (SIPP).[2]

Correlatively, it would be useful to add psychosocial and socioeconomic data to the Framingham Study and to the longitudinal components of the National Health Interview Survey (NHIS) and the National Health and Nutrition Examination Survey (NHANES).[3] The common feature of all these samples is that they are rich in either psychosocial or biomedical information but not both. A variety of possibilities need to be considered in

---

[2]The data are available electronically: National Longitudinal Survey: http://stats.bls.gov/nlshome.htm; Panel Study of Income Dynamics: http://www.isr.umich.edu/src/psid/; Health and Retirement Survey: http://www.umich.edu/~hrswww/; National Survey of Families and Households: http://www.ssc.wisc.edu/nsfh/home.htm; Survey of Income and Program Participation: http://www.sipp.census.gov/sipp/.

[3]The data are available electronically: Framingham Study: http://www.framingham.com/heart/; National Health Interview Survey: http://csa.berkeley.edu:7502/cgi.bin12/hsda?harcsda+nhis19; National Health and Nutrition Examination Survey: http://www.cdc.gov/nchs/faq/hanesii1.htm.

designating communities for inclusion in extant longitudinal studies. For example, certain people in the 1946 British birth cohort study who reside in particular settings might be designated for studies of collective community properties that influence the health of individuals. Additional people from such settings might also be enrolled in subsequent waves of the larger study. Shifting to the United States, multiple satellite studies of the National Survey of Midlife Development in the United States[4] might serve as core populations for future biobehavioral research initiatives. Similarly, the Chicago Neighborhood Study might be a critical resource for the broad-gauged investigations of pathways described herein. These specific studies are mentioned here only to illustrate the kinds of possibilities that need to be addressed. Indeed, broad consideration of communities in the United States and other countries should be part of the process of identifying the minimal set of populations to be maintained for the integrative studies delineated in this report.

Turning to animal populations, the free-ranging monkeys at Cayo Santiago Island (Berard, 1989) and Amboseli baboon communities (Altmann et al., 1993) are two instances of nonhuman primate communities that would be central resources for investigating the maintenance of allostasis, the cascade of events leading to allostatic load, and biopsychosocial pathways to diverse health outcomes. Laboratory colonies are also needed. Much more naturalistic living conditions than are currently operative—where ongoing interaction among multiple animals is facilitated—will be necessary for studies of pathway and environmentally induced gene expression delineated in Chapter 4.

CLINICAL RESEARCH CENTERS

Most major academic medical centers have a general clinical research center (GCRC) as part of their research infrastructure. The objective of these centers is to facilitate clinical studies on human populations. The emphasis, historically, in these centers has been strictly biomedical. Recently there has been encouragement for GCRC studies that integrate social and behavioral science and biomedical assessments on the same population. A prototype can be found in the GCRC at the University of Wisconsin (Ryff, 2000). A key project leading to renewed funding for that center focused on how social relationships are consequential for health. The study emerged from the growing body of research in social epidemiology, which

---

[4]The data are available electronically: National Survey of Midlife Development in the United States: http://www.pop.psu.edu/data-archive/daman/midus.html [11/27/00].

shows that those who are more socially integrated have lower profiles of disease and tend to live longer (see Chapter 5). What is poorly understood, however, is how the life-enhancing benefits of quality relationships come about. Significant others may encourage the practice of healthy behaviors, but additional influence may follow from the emotional dynamics of key relationships and how they affect underlying physiological processes. The latter mechanisms are the focus of a multidisciplinary project currently in progress at the Wisconsin GCRC. The purpose of the work, broadly defined, is to probe linkages between psychological, social, and emotional well-being and multiple aspects of biology, including allostatic load, affective neuroscience, and immune function. It is part of the larger program of characterizing predisease pathways (see Chapter 2) and pathways to positive health outcomes (see Chapter 3).

From the perspective of this report, strong bridges between community studies focusing on predisease pathways or resilience, for example, and biomedical assessments on the same population could be carried out effectively through collaborative studies with GCRCs. Ambulatory blood pressure studies with simultaneous assessment of environmental influences (Schnall et al., 1998; Pickering et al., 1996; James et al., 1991) are important prototypes for more expansive investigations linking psychosocial and biological processes. This provides a major avenue to integrate social and behavioral sciences with biology and clinical medicine, thereby fostering symbiotic relationships and greatly enriched research programs between GCRCs and the social sciences.

COMMUNITIES AND INTERVENTIONS

Health promotion and primary disease prevention intervention programs are frequently centered around communities. Thus, the selection of communities for the core population infrastructure should partially be guided by the nature of the opportunities to assess the impact of currently operative interventions as well as for implementing new ones. We also view intervention programs as opportunities to advance understanding of more basic scientific questions. For example, a program designed to enhance a sense of purpose in life among the elderly in a retirement community—with consequential downstream positive health consequences (see Chapter 3)—could be accompanied by biomarker assessments on a subset of the community with the objective of understanding the physiological substrates that underlie an improved sense of purpose in life. This kind of activity would directly improve our understanding of the biological mechanisms associated with positive health at the psychosocial level. It also points to the major opportunity to integrate intervention studies with what are typically viewed as basic research projects.

TRAINING

The multidisciplinary nature of all the thematic priorities in this report implies the need for training initiatives to support and sustain careers crossing current disciplinary boundaries. NIH has had some success in initiating and fostering such careers within biomedical disciplines. However, success in the integrative studies central to the mission of this report requires a cadre of scientists who are facile in working across multiple levels of analysis in the social, behavioral, and biomedical sciences. Linking young investigators to ongoing research of this integrative character (e.g., the recently funded mind/body centers) is one approach to developing new generations of such investigators. Training grants awarded to academic centers with a demonstrated track record of integrative research as described in this report would greatly facilitate education in the direction of "consilience" (see Chapter 1). It is of considerable importance to send clear signals that there are career paths, focused on integrative biopsychosocial topics, with promise for novel and valued scientific advancement.

RECOMMENDATIONS

NIH should provide core support for sustained infrastructure in two areas:

1. longitudinal survey populations, human communities, laboratory animal colonies, and free-ranging animal communities;
2. training initiatives to nurture and regularize the hybrid (multidisciplinary) careers of a new generation of scientists, facile in working across social, behavioral, and biomedical levels of analysis.

The vision of research proposed in this report, with its focus on the unfolding interactions between genetic, behavioral, psychosocial, and environmental factors over time and its recurrent emphasis on multilevel analysis, highlights the need for greater cross-institute strategic planning and trans-institute research initiatives. This committee has not been asked and is in no position to make detailed recommendations regarding the structure of NIH. However, the success of an integrative research approach will require collaborative efforts of the entire NIH community of scientists—medical, biological, behavioral, and social. Both incentive structures and an institutional presence will greatly facilitate such collaborative strides.

As a first step the committee recommends that NIH create an internal mechanism for developing consensus on the most promising research opportunities within and across the thematic priorities, as well as a locus for strategic planning for future trans-institute initiatives.

REFERENCES

Altmann J, Schoeller D, Altmann S, Muruthi P, Sapolsky R. 1993 "Body size and fatness of free-living baboons reflect food availability and activity levels" *American Journal of Primatology* 30:149-161.

Berard JD. 1989 "A four-year study of the association between male dominance rank, residency status and reproductive activity in rhesus macaques *(macaca mulatta)*" *Primates* 40:163-178.

Berkman LF, Breslow L. 1983 *Health and Ways of Living: The Alameda County Study* (New York: Oxford University Press).

Dawber T. 1980 *The Framingham Study* (Cambridge MA: Harvard University Press).

Hauser RM, Carr D, Hauser T, Hayes J, Krecker M, Hsiang-Hui DK, Magee W, Presti J, Shinberg D, Sweeney M, Thompson-Colon T, Uhrig SCN, Warren JR. 1993 *The Class of 1957 After 35 Years: Overview and Preliminary Findings* Working paper No. 93-17 for the Center for Demography and Ecology, University of Wisconsin, Madison.

James GD, Moucha OP, Pickering TG. 1991 "The normal hourly variation of blood pressure in women: Average patterns and the effect of work strain" *Journal of Human Hypertension* 5:505-509.

National Institute on Aging. 1991 *Research on Older Women and Highlights from the Baltimore Longitudinal Study of Aging* (Bethesda MD: U.S. Department of Health and Human Services).

Pickering TG, Devereux RB, James GD, Gerin W, Landsbergis P, Schnall PL, Schwartz JE. 1996 "Environmental influences on blood pressure and the role of job strain" *Journal of Hypertension* 14/suppl.J:S179-S185.

Power C, Matthews S. 1998 "Accumulation of health risks across social groups in a national longitudinal study" in Strickland SS, Shetty PS (eds.). *Human Biology and Social Inequality* (Cambridge U.K.: Cambridge University Press) 36-57.

Russek LG, Schwartz GE. 1997 "Feelings of parental caring predict health status in midlife: A 35-year follow-up of the Harvard Mastery of Stress Study" *Journal of Behavioral Medicine* 20:1-13.

Ryff CD. 2000 "How are social relationships consequential for health?" *The Link*, a publication of the University of Wisconsin-Madison General Clinical Research Center 4:1-2.

Sampson RJ, Raudenbush SW, Earls F. 1997 "Neighborhoods and violent crime: A multilevel study of collective efficacy" *Science* 227/5328:918-924.

Schnall PL, Schwartz JE, Landsbergis PA, Warren K, Pickering TG. 1998 "A longitudinal study of job strain and ambulatory blood pressure: Results from a three-year follow-up" *Psychosomatic Medicine* 60/6:697-706.

Wadsworth MEJ, Kuh DJL. 1997 "Childhood influences on adult health: A review of recent work from the British 1946 national birth cohort study, the MRC National Survey of Health and Development" *Pediatric Perinatal Epidemiology* 11:2-20.

Biographical Sketches

BURTON H. SINGER (*Chair*) is professor of demography and public affairs at the Woodrow Wilson School, Princeton University. Dr. Singer's work has altered the ways in which quantitative studies of economic, social, and epidemiological processes are carried out to determine causal mechanisms and associations. His research interests include the epidemiology of tropical diseases, demography and economics of aging, health and social consequences of economic development, and the interrelationships between genetics and historical demography. At Yale University he served as chair of the Department of Epidemiology and Public Health. He was elected to the National Academy of Sciences in 1994 and was a Guggenheim fellow in 1981-1982. Dr. Singer has served as chair of several National Research Council (NRC) committees.

LISA F. BERKMAN is chair of the Department of Health and Social Behavior and is Norman Professor of Health and Social Behavior and of Epidemiology at the Harvard School of Public Health. She is also chair of the Harvard Center for Society and Health. Dr. Berkman is an epidemiologist whose research focuses on social influences on health outcomes and their role in predicting declines in physical and cognitive functioning and the onset of disease and mortality. She is particularly interested in the role of social networks, social integration, and social inequalities and health. She serves as chair of the Steering Committee on Enhanced Recovery in Coronary Heart Disease of the National Heart, Lung, and Blood Institute (NHLBI). She has been a member of the Advisory Board for the NHLBI study of cardiovascular disease in the elderly. She serves on the IOM Committee on Health and Behavior: Research Practices and Policy.

LINDA M. BURTON is director of the Center for Human Development and Family Research in Diverse Contexts and professor of human development and family studies and sociology at Pennsylvania State University. Her research explores the relationship of neighborhood contexts, poverty, intergenerational family processes, and mental health outcomes across the life course. She is currently involved in a four-year multisite collaborative study of the impact of welfare reform on families and children. Dr. Burton has been a Spencer Foundation fellow, a Brookdale National fellow, and a fellow at the Center for Advanced Study in the Behavioral Sciences, Stanford, California. In 1996 she received the American Family Therapy Academy Award for innovative contributions to family research, the Faculty Medal for Outstanding Achievement of Pennsylvania State University, and a "Products of Compton" Award. She currently serves on the Board on Behavioral, Cognitive, and Sensory Sciences for the NRC and is director of the Research Consortium on Diversity, Family Processes, and Child Adolescent Mental Health as well as the consortium's multisite postdoctoral training program, which are sponsored by the National Institute of Mental Health.

JOHN T. CACIOPPO is the Tiffany and Margaret Blake Distinguished Service Professor at the University of Chicago, directs the social psychology program, and is a member of the executive committee of the Institute for Mind and Biology. Dr. Cacioppo has also served as chaired university professor of psychology at Ohio State University, as director of the National Science Foundation-sponsored Program for advanced study and research in social psychophysiology, and as director of the National Institute of Mental Health-sponsored social psychology training program grant at Ohio State University. Dr. Cacioppo has been a Sigma Xi national lecturer, president of the Society for Psychophysiological Research, president for the Society for Consumer Research, and president of the Society for Personality and Social Psychology, and a member of the Board of Directors for the Ohio State University Research Foundation. He is the recipient of the Distinguished Scientific Award for an Early Career Contribution to Psychophysiology, the National Academy of Sciences Troland Research Award, and numerous other awards. Dr. Cacioppo is the former editor in chief of *Psychophysiology*, a former associate editor of *Psychological Review*, and a former member of the John D. and Catherine T. MacArthur Foundation Research Network on Mind/Body Interactions. He has been elected to the Society of Experimental Social Psychology and the Gesellschaft fur Unendliche Versuche and is a fellow in the Society for Personality and Social Psychology, American Psychological Association, Academy of Behavioral Medicine Research, International Organization of Psychophysiology, American Psychological Society, American Association for the Advancement of Science, and the Society for Behavioral Medicine.

MARGARET A. CHESNEY is professor of medicine at the University of California at San Francisco. She is nationally recognized as an expert in behavioral medicine with a focus on interventions for prevention and coping with chronic disease. She received her Ph.D. from Colorado State University and was a postdoctoral fellow in psychiatry at the School of Medicine, Temple University. Dr. Chesney is codirector of the Center for AIDS Prevention Studies and a senior scientist involved in several projects studying behavioral factors in the prevention and treatment of HIV disease. In addition, she is director of the behavioral core of the Center for AIDS Research at San Francisco General Hospital and associate director of the California AIDS Research Center at UCSF. Prior to joining the University of California, she was director of the Department of Behavioral Medicine at Stanford Research Institute. Margaret Chesney currently serves on the IOM Board on Neuroscience and Behavioral Health and is past president of the Division of Health Psychology of the American Psychological Association, the American Psychosomatic Society, and the Academy of Behavioral Medicine Research.

DAVID CUTLER is the John L. Loeb Professor of Social Sciences of the Department of Economics and the Kennedy School of Government of Harvard University. He received his Ph.D. from MIT in 1991 and his A.B., summa cum laude, from Harvard in 1987. He is affiliated with the National Bureau of Economic Research, the Employee Benefit Research Institute, and the Institute for Research on Policy and serves as the editor or associate editor of several economic journals. Dr. Cutler served on the NRC Committee on the NIH Research Priority-Setting Process. Dr. Cutler is the editor of the *Journal of Health Economics* and associate editor of the *Journal of Public Economics*.

BARUCH FISCHHOFF is university professor in the Departments of Social and Decision Sciences and of Engineering and Public Policy at Carnegie Mellon University. He holds a B.S. in mathematics from Wayne State University and an M.A. and a Ph.D. in psychology from the Hebrew University of Jerusalem. He is a fellow of the American Psychological Association and a recipient of its Early Career Awards for Distinguished Scientific Contribution to Psychology and for Contributions to Psychology in the Public Interest. He is a fellow of the Society for Risk Analysis as well as a recipient of its Distinguished Achievement Award. His current research includes risk communication, adolescent decision making, evaluation of environmental damages, medical informed consent, and insurance-related behavior. He serves on the editorial boards of several journals, including *Journal of Risk and Uncertainty* and *Journal of Experimental Psychology: Applied*. Dr. Fischhoff is a member of the IOM.

JEROME KAGAN is the Daniel and Amy Starch Professor of Psychology at Harvard University. He has taught at Harvard since 1964. At the present time Professor Kagan's laboratory is devoted to the biological/biomedical study of temperamental qualities in young children with a focus on two specific groups called inhibited and uninhibited. Professor Kagan took his A.B. at Rutgers University and his Ph.D. at Yale University. After a faculty appointment at Ohio State University and service in the U.S. Army he went to the Fels Research Institute in Yellow Springs, Ohio. A major project at the institute involved evaluation of a group of adults who had been followed by the staff of the institute since they were young children. Dr. Kagan is a recipient of the Distinguished Scientist Award of the American Psychological Association. In 1987 he was elected to the IOM and has served on two NRC committees.

BRUCE S. McEWEN is professor and head of the laboratory of neuroendocrinology at Rockefeller University. A major figure in behavioral neuroendocrinology, Dr. McEwen has produced a massive body of important work on the roles of steroid hormones in reproductive behavior, brain development, gene expression in the brain, and brain plasticity in adulthood and on the effects of stress on the age-related brain degeneration that causes cognitive deficits. He is a past president of the Society for Neuroscience and a member of the Endocrine Society and American Society for Neurochemistry, among other organizations. He is a member of the Research Network for Socioeconomic Status and Health of the John D. and Catherine T. MacArthur Foundation. Dr. McEwen was elected to the National Academy of Sciences in 1997 and the IOM in 1998 and has served on several NRC and IOM committees.

BARBARA J. McNEIL is the Ridley Watts Professor and head of the Department of Health Care Policy at Harvard Medical School and professor of radiology at Harvard Medical School and the Brigham and Women's Hospital. Dr. McNeil received her bachelor's degree in chemistry from Emmanuel College, her M.D. from Harvard Medical School, and her Ph.D. in biochemistry from Harvard University. After interning in pediatrics at the Massachusetts General Hospital, she trained in nuclear medicine at Harvard Medical School. She was the founding head of the Department of Health Care Policy at Harvard Medical School in 1988. She continues to practice nuclear medicine at the Brigham and Women's Hospital. Dr. McNeil is a member of the national Blue Cross Technology Assessment Commission and the Council for Performance Measurement for the Joint Commission on Accreditation of Healthcare Organizations. She has served on the IOM Governing Board. Currently, she is vice-chair of the IOM's Board on Health Care Services and is a member of the NRC Commission on Behavioral and Social Sciences and Education. Dr. McNeil is a member of the publications committee of the Massachusetts Medical Society, publisher of the *New England Journal of Medicine.* She continues to be active in several national groups in radiology and nuclear medicine, including the National Council on Radiation Protection. Dr. McNeil's research has involved several broad areas related to the effectiveness and quality of medical practice. She directed one of the first patient outcome research teams funded by the Agency for Health Care Policy Research and is now the principal investigator of a successor project to help improve the care of Medicare beneficiaries after a heart attack. Her work in technology assessment involves imaging technologies. She has recently established a group of several national managed care organizations to implement and evaluate a series of quality measures for patients with cardiac disease.

MICHAEL J. MEANEY is professor of psychiatry at McGill University, with his laboratory situated at the Douglas Hospital Research Center. Dr. Meaney's research focuses on the development of individual differences in behavioral and endocrine responses to stress and their importance in determining vulnerability/resistance to stress-induced illness. The research approaches range in scope from molecular biology to human clinical studies. Dr. Meaney has been awarded a University Research Fellowship (Natural Sciences and Engineering Research Council of Canada), as well as scientist and senior scientist awards (from the Medical Research Council of Canada). He is on the editorial board of *Hormones and Behavior, Behavioral Neuroscience,* and the *Journal of Neuroendocrinology.* Research in Dr. Meaney's laboratory has developed through collaborations with individuals such as Drs. Jonathan Seckl, Robert Sapolsky, Paul Plotsky, Remi Quirion, and Greg Rose, as well as the continued mentorship of Bruce McEwen. Michael Meaney was educated in his native Montreal, obtaining an undergraduate degree from Loyola College and a Ph.D. from Concordia University under the supervision of Jane Stewart. He was a postdoctoral fellow in neuroendocrinology with Bruce McEwen at the Rockefeller University and subsequently returned to Montreal.

CAROL D. RYFF is director of the Institute on Aging and professor of psychology at the University of Wisconsin-Madison. She is a member of the MacArthur Research Network of Successful Midlife Development, a fellow of the American Psychological Association and the Gerontological Society of America, a former fellow at the Center for Advanced Study in the Behavioral Sciences at Stanford, and consulting editor for the *Journal of Personality and Social Psychology* and *Psychology and Aging.* She has catalyzed extensive multidisciplinary research via conferences and edited volumes. Her work has been supported by the National Institute on Aging, the National Institute of Mental Health, and the MacArthur Foundation. Dr. Ryff's research centers on the study of psychological well-being, an area in which she has generated a theory-driven, empirically based approach to assessment of multiple dimensions of positive psychological functioning.

These assessment procedures have been translated into 17 languages and are used in diverse studies in the fields of psychology, sociology, demography, epidemiology, and health. Her own descriptive studies, conducted with nationally representative survey samples, have documented socio-demographic correlates of well-being (i.e., how positive mental health varies by age, gender, social class, ethnic/minority status). Explanatory studies have focused on individuals' life experiences and their interpretations of them to account for variations in well-being. Longitudinal investigations of midlife development and old age explore processes of resilience and vulnerability via the cumulation of adversity and advantage. Multiple protective factors (biological, psychological, social) hypothesized to promote resilience are currently under investigation. The linkages between positive mental health and positive physical health are a primary focus in ongoing longitudinal studies.

ROBERT J. SAMPSON is Lucy Flower Professor of Sociology at the University of Chicago and a research fellow at the American Bar Foundation. His major research interests include criminology, the life course, and community/urban sociology. Dr. Sampson is currently studying the sources and consequences of community-level social organization (e.g., collective efficacy, social capital, network density, organizational participation) as part of the Project on Human Development in Chicago Neighborhoods, for which he serves as scientific director. He is also engaged in a longitudinal study of crime and deviance over 70 years in the lives of 1,000 disadvantaged men born in Boston during the Great Depression. His recent book with John Laub on this project, *Crime in the Making: Pathways and Turning Points Through Life* (Harvard University Press, 1993), received the outstanding book award from the American Society of Criminology, the Academy of Criminal Justice Sciences, and the Crime, Law, and Deviance Section of the American Sociological Association. In 1997 Dr. Sampson was a fellow at the Center for Advanced Study in the Behavioral Sciences, Stanford, California. In 1994 he was named fellow of the American Society of Criminology. Dr. Sampson previously served with a NRC work group on communities and crime.

SHELLEY E. TAYLOR is a professor of psychology at the University of California, Los Angeles. She received her Ph.D. from Yale University in 1972 and joined the Harvard Faculty of Psychology and Social Relations, where she remained until 1979. At UCLA she has chaired the Social Psychology Program (1990-1994) and has chaired or cochaired the health psychology program continuously since 1979. Dr. Taylor is the recipient of the Early Career Award from the American Psychological Association, the Donald Campbell Award in Social Psychology, the Distinguished Scientific Contribution Award in Health Psychology, and the American Psychological Association's Distinguished Scientist Award. Her research program addresses self-regulatory and social processes in the management of stress and the role of psychosocial variables in the progression of disease, especially cancer and AIDS. Her current work explores the interplay of biology and psychology and its role in affecting mental health and health outcomes across the life span.

DAVID R. WILLIAMS is a professor of sociology and senior research scientist in the Institute for Social Research at the University of Michigan. His previous academic appointment was at Yale University. Dr. Williams's research has focused on differences in socioeconomic status in health in general and the health of the African American population in particular. He has served as a consultant to numerous federal health agencies and private organizations. He has also served on the National Committee on Vital and Health Statistics and chaired its Subcommittee on Minority and Other Special Populations. He is a member of the National Science Foundation's Board of Overseers for the General Social Survey. He has an M.P.H. from Loma Linda University, a M.Div. from Andrews University, and a Ph.D. in sociology from the University of Michigan. He has served on the NRC Panel on Needle Exchange and Bleach Distribution Programs.

Index

A

Accidents and injuries, 29, 50, 92, 93, 95, 97, 106, 129
Adolescents, 29
    alcohol and drug use, 129
    contraceptive use, 138
    delinquent behavior, 35
    depression, 137
    diabetes, 37
    personal ties, 36, 54, 74-75
    positive health, 52, 54
    predisease pathways, 29, 34-35, 36, 37
    pregnancy, 138-139
    sexually transmitted diseases, 122, 138-139
    smoking, 34-35, 128
    socioeconomic status, 104
Adrenal gland, 33, 45, 80, 168
    epinephrine, 27, 37, 39, 80, 172, 174
    norepinephrine, 27, 37, 66, 74, 172, 174
    see also Hypothalamic-pituitary-adrenal (HPA) axis
African Americans, *see* Black persons
Age factors, 4, 45
    alcohol abuse, 129
    cumulative risk and aging, 27
    diet, 139
    disability/disease onset, 2, 5, 10, 46, 47, 48, 64, 81, 131, 134, 136, 149, 165
    gene expression in midlife, 65-66
    fertility, 135
    midlife, 65-66, 105
    personal ties, 74
    smoking, 128
    temperament, 34
    see also Adolescents; Children; Elderly persons; Infants; Life expectancy; Pregnancy and prenatal development
AIDS, *see* HIV/AIDS
Alameda County Study, 105, 185
Alcohol and drug use, 34, 35, 129
    adolescents, 129
    community-level factors, 92
    interventions, 35, 151
    mother-child relations, 30
    positive health, 52
    pregnancy and prenatal development, 35
    racial/ethnic factors, 106
    social factors, 36
    time horizons, 4, 22, 40
Allostasis and allostatic load, 4, 5, 6, 7, 12, 18, 46, 70, 126, 172-175, 186, 187
    gender factors, 174-175
    personal ties, 83-84

predisease pathways, 20, 26-27, 35-40
race/ethnicity, 97
socioeconomic status and, 48-49, 103, 104
Alternative medicine, 141-142, 144
Alzheimer's disease, *see* Dementia
American Indians, *see* Native Americans
Amino acid regulation, 32
Animal models, 179
    colony infrastructure, 6, 13, 70, 184,
        186, 188
    environmentally induced gene
        expression, 6, 66-69, 70, 77
    environmental stressors, 33, 37
    exercise and neurogenesis, 169
    intergenerational transmission of
        behavior, 67-68
    mother-child behavior, 28-30, 31, 32,
        66-69, 77, 78-79
    personal ties, 7, 76, 77, 84
    positive health, 46-47, 169-170
    recovery from disease, 33
    self-efficacy and recovery from disease, 33
    social relations, 6, 7, 13, 76, 77, 84,
        170, 184, 186; *see also "personal
        ties" above*
    socioeconomic hierarchies, 9, 103
    substance abuse during pregnancy, 35
Anxiety, 31, 32, 33, 50, 142
Asians and Pacific Islanders, 107, 110
Assessment, *see* Research infrastructure;
        Research methodology
Asset and Health Dynamics Survey, 133
Asthma, 10, 126, 134-135, 143, 148
Attitudes
    stigmatization, 3, 9, 23-29, 107, 109-
        110, 111, 155
    toward cancer and HIV patients, 155
    see also Emotional factors; Racism and
        discrimination

B

Baltimore Longitudinal Study of Aging, 185
Behavior, individual, 1-2, 17-18, 20, 40, 188
    community-level factors, 91
    cumulative risk, 26
    gene expression, 64, 129-130, 149
    intergenerational transfer, 30, 31, 34,
        67-68
    interventions, general, 11, 12, 149-152,
        156, 160; *see also* Health
        promotion

personal ties, 74-75, 82
population surveys, 10, 11, 118, 143
positive health, 5, 47, 52-53, 56, 57
predisease pathways, 3-4, 25, 32, 34-36,
    176-177
primary prevention, 52-53
research methodology, 176-177, 179, 180
socioeconomic hierarchies, 9, 102-103
see also Alcohol and drug use; Exercise;
        Mental illness; Nutrition;
        Personal ties; Primary prevention;
        Psychological factors; Sexually
        transmitted diseases; Smoking;
        Social factors
Benzodiazapine system, 32
Birth cohorts, *see* Cohort studies
Birth weight, 36, 65, 91, 92, 93, 96, 119,
    125, 134, 138
Black persons, 106, 108-111
    mortality, 106, 108, 110
    occupational hazards, 108
Brain function and structure, 171-172, 173
    child-mother interactions, 29
    hippocampus, 26, 77
    historical perspectives, 17
    medulla, 29, 31, 33, 168
        epinephrine, 27, 37, 39, 80, 172, 174
        norepinephrine, 27, 37, 66, 74, 172,
            174
    personal ties, 7, 73, 77-79, 84
    positive health, 46-47, 171
    prenatal development, 28
Breast cancer, 35, 50, 75, 129, 155
Britain, *see* United Kingdom

C

Cancer, 173
    attitudes toward patients, 155
    breast, 35, 50, 75, 129, 155
    diet, 129
    early childhood experiences and, 29
    genomics, 69-70, 155
    interventions, general, 151, 157
    lung, 22, 75, 126, 132
    National Cancer Act, 1, 19
    National Cancer Institute, 1, 19, 45,
        157-158
    ovarian, 155
    personal ties, 75, 151-153
    population-level health, 129, 131
    positive health, 52

psychological factors, 151, 155
race/ethnicity and, 106, 107, 108
recovery, 33, 75
Cardiovascular disease, 25, 130-131, 148,
149, 173
community-level factors, 95
cost of interventions, 139-140, 152
cumulative risk, 26, 27
diet, 129, 130-131, 139
emotional regulation and, 33
interventions, 139-140, 148, 149, 152
parenting and, 29
personal ties, 76, 83
positive health, 50, 52
psychological factors, 1, 33, 34, 38, 50,
76, 152
racial/ethnic factors, 106, 108-109
recovery from, 50
smoking, 22, 140
social factors, 22; *see also "personal
ties" above*
socioeconomic status, 101, 106
see also Hypertension; National Heart,
Lung, and Blood Institute
Catecholamines, 32, 74, 77
Centers for Disease Control and Prevention
(CDC), 122, 134
Child-mother interactions, 28-31, 68-69,
76, 77, 143
alcohol abuse, 30
animal models, 28-30, 31, 32, 66-69,
77, 78-79
brain development, 29
environmentally induced gene
expression, 29-30, 32, 66-68
immune response, 77
socioeconomic status and, 103
Children, 45, 167-168, 174
asthma, 10, 126, 134-135, 143, 148
cancer, 29
chronic diseases and disabilities, 10, 29,
126, 127
developing countries, 135, 136
disabled, parents of, 126
divorce, effects on, 52, 74
early life experiences, 4-5, 6, 22, 28-32,
39-40, 103, 104, 133, 167-168
genetic factors, 29-30
genomics, 134-135
interventions, 153
longitudinal studies, 133
mental illness, 51

obesity, 153
personal ties, 73-75; *see also* Parents and
parenting
population-level health, 10, 118-119,
125-126, 133, 134-135, 136, 168
resilience, 48
school-based interventions, 11, 54
socioeconomic status, 48, 103, 104, 134
see also Adolescents; Birth weight;
Infants; Pregnancy and prenatal
development
Cholesterol, 25, 27, 33, 51, 139-140, 149,
153, 165, 173
Chronic disease and disability, 45, 168-169
alternative medicine therapies, 142
childhood, 10, 29, 126, 127
elderly persons, 120, 130, 131, 132,
136-137
interventions, general, 11, 151
onset of, 2, 5, 10, 46, 47, 48, 64, 81,
131, 134, 136, 149, 165
pain and pain management, 50, 127,
142, 148, 151, 152
population-level health, 119-121, 126,
127, 130-133
psychological factors, 34
quality of life, 51
socioeconomic status, 101, 131-132
*see also specific diseases and body
systems*
Cities, *see* Urban areas
Clinical practice guidelines, 36
Cognitive factors, 169
cumulative risk, 26
mind/body centers, 2, 19, 55, 142, 188
personal ties, 74
positive health, 50, 52
predisease pathways, 26, 32
recovery from disease, 50
social relationships, 22, 74
socioeconomic status, 104
see also Educational attainment
Cohort studies, 13, 104-106, 110, 130,
165-167, 172, 185, 186
Communicable disease, *see* Immune system
and infectious diseases
Community-level factors, 3, 8, 18, 23, 91-
99, 143
alcohol and drug use, 92
children, 48
interventions, general, 11, 13, 91, 153-
154, 156, 158, 187

longitudinal studies, 8, 92, 98, 105, 143,
    185-186
positive health, 5, 8, 57
prediscase pathways, 2, 39, 97
racial segregation, 9, 92, 93, 108, 111
research infrastructure, 13, 185-186,
    187, 188
    animal colonies, 6, 13, 70, 184, 186,
        188
research methodology, 8, 95-97, 98,
    164, 170
resilience, 48
socioeconomic status, 92-95, 97-98,
    102-103, 106, 108
    see also Rural areas; Urban areas
Comorbidity, 20, 27
    community-level factors, 92
    mental illness, 51
Contraceptive use, 138
Co-occurring risk factors, see Allostasis and
    allostatic load
Corticotropin-releasing hormone (CRH),
    37, 66
Cortisol, 32, 74, 76, 172
Cost and cost-benefit factors, 158, 167
    adolescents, contraceptives, 138-139
    adolescents, smoking cessation, 150
    alternative medicine therapies, 142, 144
    asthma, 143
    cardiovascular disease interventions,
        139-140, 152
    cholesterol therapy, 139
    community-level interventions, 91
    disabled children, parents of, 126, 143
    elderly, care of, 136-137
    health promotion, 138-139
    managed care, 10, 140-141, 144
    medical interventions, 138, 139-140,
        142, 144, 152; see also Health
        insurance
    nutrition interventions, 53
    population-level health, 126, 136-137,
        139-140, 142, 143, 144, 153-154
    tobacco tax, 150, 154, 157
Council of Public Representatives (COPR),
    14-15, 53, 56
    committee study methodology, xii, 14
Crime and criminal behavior, 8, 92, 108,
    129
    adolescent delinquence, 35
    homicide, 91, 92, 95, 106

smoking laws, 154
suicide, 29, 92, 106, 110, 111
    see also Alcohol and drug abuse
Cultural factors, 10, 17, 52, 75, 92, 93-94,
    97, 111
    language, 73-74
    religion, 111
    violence, 8, 94
    see also Social factors

D

Dementia, 39, 65, 77, 80, 165, 173
Demographic and Health Surveys, 119
Demographic factors
    migration, 110
    see also Age factors; Community-level
        factors; Educational attainment;
        Elderly persons; Gender factors;
        Population health; Race/ethnicity;
        Rural areas; Socioeconomic
        status; Urban areas
Depression, 29, 32, 33, 34, 40, 45, 105,
    137, 142, 171
Developing countries, 101, 135, 136
Diabetes, 26, 36, 37, 48, 106, 130-131, 148
Diet, see Nutrition
Differential survival processes, 5, 8, 49, 50,
    82, 101
Disabilities and disabled persons, see
    Chronic disease and disability
Discrimination, see Racism and
    discrimination
Dopamine regulation, 32, 34, 35
Drug use, see Alcohol and drug use

E

Eating disorders, 9, 75, 148, 152, 156, 157
Economic factors
    population health and macroeconomy,
        10, 106, 118, 131-132, 135-137,
        143-144
    see also Cost and cost-benefit factors;
        Employment and unemployment;
        Funding; Socioeconomic status;
        Taxation, tobacco
Education, see Health promotion;
    Professional education; Public
    education

Educational attainment, 9, 100, 101, 102, 107, 108, 111, 132
  smoking, 128
Elderly persons, 10, 45, 165, 169, 174-175, 187
  chronic diseases and disabilities, 120, 130, 131, 132, 136-137
  comorbidity, 27
  dementia, 39, 65, 77, 80, 165, 173
  disabled, 120
  female family caregivers of, 39
  gender factors, 39, 174-175
  resilience, 55
  self-efficacy, 32-33
  temperament, 34
  personal ties, 74
Emotional factors, 5, 7, 84, 179
  anxiety, 31, 32, 33, 50, 142
  cancer, 75
  depression, 29, 32, 33, 34, 40, 45, 105, 137, 142, 171
  disabled children, parents of, 126
  neurological factors, 33, 77-78
  positive health, 50-51, 52, 54-55
  recovery from disease, 50-51, 75
  regulation of emotions, predisease pathways, 29, 30, 32, 33
  see also Personal ties
Employment and unemployment, 8, 9, 38-39, 100, 102, 103, 111, 168-169
  cancer/HIV patients, discrimination, 155
  disabled children, parents of, 126
  fertility and, 135
  gender factors, 38-39, 133
  interventions, worksite, 11, 154, 158
  positive health, 11, 52
  race/ethnicity, 108
Environmental factors, general, 3, 11-15 (passim), 17, 21, 22, 45, 126
  animal models, 6, 33, 37, 66-69, 70, 77
  gene expression, 3, 6, 17-18, 23, 26, 29-30, 32, 40, 63-72, 76, 77, 166, 172
    animal models, 6, 66-69, 70, 77
    children, 29-30, 32, 66-68
  population-level health, 10, 118
  positive health, 5, 54, 56
  predisease pathways, 4, 36-39, 25-26, 32, 36-39, 97
  resistance and resilience, 48
  see also Community-level factors; Social factors

Environmental Genome Project, 134-135
Epidemiology, 22
  personal ties, 7, 75, 76, 82
  see also Longitudinal studies; Mortality; Population health
Epinephrine, 27, 37, 39, 80, 172, 174
Ethnicity, see Race/ethnicity; Racism and discrimination
Europe, 101-102, 105
  see also United Kingdom
Exercise, 34, 35, 46-47, 52, 129, 139, 149, 151, 152, 169

F

Familial factors, 14, 38, 74-75, 83
  dementia, caregivers, 39, 65, 77, 80
  interventions, 11, 152-153, 156
  predisease pathways, 4, 25-26
  working women, 38-39
  see also Child-mother interactions; Children; Marriage and marital status; Parents and parenting
Federal government
  Centers for Disease Control and Prevention (CDC), 122, 134
  health insurance, 138; see also Medicare
  tobacco tax, 150, 154, 157
  toxic waste regulations, 132
  see also Funding; Legislation; terms with "National Institute"
Females, see Gender factors
Fertility, 135
Foreign countries, see International perspectives
Framingham Study, 105, 143, 185
Funding, 179, 188
  historical perspectives, 1, 19
  interventions, general, 158
  social factors, 186-187
  socioeconomic status research, 104-105
  see also Research infrastructure

G

Gender factors
  adolescent sexual activity, 138-139
  allostatic load, 174-175
  cancer risk, 47-48
  chronic disease, 130

diet, 139
elderly, caregivers of, 39
elderly persons, 174-175
employment, 38-39, 133
HIV, optimism among male patients, 50
life expectancy, 136
personal ties, 74, 75, 83
recovery from disease, 50
sexually transmitted diseases, 133
smoking, 34, 128
see also Breast cancer; Child-mother
        interactions; Ovarian cancer;
        Pregnancy and prenatal
        development
Genetics, 47-48
behavioral risk factors, general, 64, 129-
        130, 149
cancer risk, 47
cumulative risk and, 26
diabetes, 48
emotional regulation, 33
environmentally induced gene
        expression, 3, 6, 17-18, 23, 26,
        29-30, 32, 40, 63-72, 76, 77,
        166, 172
    animal models, 6, 66-69, 70, 77
    children, 29-30, 32, 66-68
historical perspectives, 17
hypertension, 47-48, 67-68
intergenerational transfer of behaviors,
        30, 31, 34, 67-68
microarray chip technologies, 6, 64, 70,
        166
mother-child interactions and, 29-30
personal ties and, 7, 29, 65-66, 76, 77, 84
positive health, 5, 53, 57
predisease pathways, 4-5, 26, 28, 32,
        155
time horizons, 22
Genomics, 45, 69-70, 64, 69-70, 155
allostatic load, 175
cancer, 69-70, 155
child health, 134-135
personal ties, 74
prenatal development, 28
Geographic information systems, 97
Going for the Goal (GOAL) program, 54
Gonorrhea, 121-122

H

Harvard Mastery of Stress Study, 185
Health and Retirement Survey, 133, 185
Health care, *see* Medical interventions
Health insurance, 133, 138, 143
managed care, 10, 140-141, 144
Medicare, 133, 137, 140
Health promotion, 1, 5, 11, 12, 19, 148
adolescents, 54
cholesterol reduction, 139-140, 149, 153
cost of, 138-139
research infrastructure, 13, 45
smoking prevention, 35
see also Public education
Heart disease, *see* Cardiovascular disease
Hippocampus, 26, 77
Hispanics, 106, 107, 108, 110, 111
Historical perspectives, 17, 19, 21, 22
alternative medicine therapies, 141-142
chronic diseases, 130-131
communicable disease, 123-125
disability rates, 120-121
life expectancy, 17, 119, 120, 130-131
medical interventions, 17, 130, 138
nutrition, 130-131
personal ties and autonomic activity, 79
racism, 107
socioeconomic status, 100-101
substance abuse, 129
HIV/AIDS, 28, 50, 108, 122, 123, 129,
        148, 152, 153, 155, 157
Homicide, 91, 92, 95, 106
HPA axis, *see* Hypothalamic-pituitary-
        adrenal (HPA) axis
Hypertension, 25, 131, 165
cost-effectiveness of preventive
        interventions, 139-140
cumulative risk, 26
genetic factors, 47-48, 67-68
intergenerational transfer of behavior,
        67-68
occupational stress and, 38, 39
parents and children, 33
personal ties, 75, 76
psychological factors, 1, 33, 38
social isolation, 75
Hypothalamic-pituitary-adrenal (HPA) axis,
        26, 27, 31, 46, 70, 76, 77, 80, 168

I

Immigration and immigrants, 110
see also Asians and Pacific Islanders;
Hispanics
Immune system and infectious diseases, 169,
172
children, 77
chronic stress, 6, 37
cumulative risk, 26
personal ties, 65-66, 77, 79-82, 84
population-level health, 118, 121-125,
132, 133-134
positive health, 55
psychological factors, 33-34, 151
tuberculosis, 108, 121, 123-125, 134
see also Neurological factors; Sexually
transmitted diseases; *specific
diseases*
Indians, see Native Americans
Infants, 12
birth weight, 36, 65, 91, 92, 93, 96,
119, 125, 134, 138
mortality, 91, 92, 93, 119, 125, 130,
134, 135
see also Child-mother interactions
Infectious disease, see Immune system and
infectious diseases
Injuries, see Accidents and injuries
Insurance, see Health insurance; Managed
care
Inter-American Development Bank, 135-136
Interdisciplinary approaches
committee study at hand, 19, 20
see also Multidisciplinary approaches
International perspectives
chronic disease and disability, 120-121
cultural factors, 75, 102
life expectancy, 119, 120, 131, 135, 136
macroeconomic effects, 135
medical interventions, 137, 138
mortality, 135, 136
population health, 119, 120-121, 123,
131, 135-136, 153-154, 165-166,
185-186
quality of life, 119
racism, 108
sexually transmitted disease, 122
socioeconomic status, 101-102, 104-
105, 119, 130, 131, 135-136
tuberculosis, 123

Interventions, general, 2, 3, 11-12, 24, 148-
163, 178-179, 187-188
alcohol and substance abuse, 35, 151
cancer, 151, 157
cardiovascular disease, 139-140, 148,
149, 152
children, 153
chronic diseases and disabilities, 11, 151
community-level factors, 11, 13, 91,
153-154, 156, 158, 187
immigration and immigrants, 110
individual behavior, 11, 12, 149-152,
156, 160
longitudinal studies, 159, 166-167
multidisciplinary, 11, 12, 178-179, 187
nutrition, 53, 149, 151
pain and pain management, 50, 127,
142, 148, 151, 152
population health, 149, 153-154, 158
psychological factors, 11, 12, 148-149,
151-152, 156, 160
school-based, 11, 54
smoking, 35, 128, 148, 150-151, 154, 157
social, 36-37
weight control, 35
worksite, 11, 154, 158
see also Exercise; Health promotion;
Medical interventions; Primary
prevention; Public education

K

Kaiser Family Foundation, 121(n.2)

L

Language factors, 73-74
Legislation
managed care, 140
National Cancer Act, 1, 19
Life expectancy, 2, 17, 118, 119, 120, 130-
131, 136, 148
see also Mortality
Local factors, see Community-level factors
Longitudinal studies, 5, 12, 13, 40, 133,
143, 174, 185, 188
children, 133
cohort studies, 13, 104-106, 110, 130,
165-167, 172, 185, 186

community-level factors, 8, 92, 98, 105, 143, 185-186
co-occurring risk factors, 12, 27
interventions, 159, 166-167
occupational stress, 38
personal ties, 7, 8, 27, 84
positive health, 12, 13, 49, 51-52, 56
predisease pathways, 4, 40, 56, 165-167, 185
racism and discrimination, 109-110
socioeconomic hierarchies, 9-10, 102, 104-106, 109-110, 111
see also Population health; *specific studies and surveys*
Lung cancer, 22, 75, 126, 132

M

MacArthur Study of Successful Aging, 165
Malaysian Life History Survey, 105
Males, *see* Gender factors
Managed care, 10, 140-141, 144
Marriage and marital status, 36, 74, 83
divorce and marital conflict, 31, 52, 74
recovery from disease, 75
Maternal factors, *see* Child-mother interactions
Medical interventions, 11, 132-133, 137-142, 143, 144, 148, 160, 186-187
alternative medicine therapies, 141-142, 144
behavioral interventions integrated with, 156
cost factors, 138, 139-140, 142, 144, 152; *see also* Health insurance
disabled children, parents of, 126
historical perspectives, 17, 130, 138
international perspectives, 137, 138
population studies, 11, 118, 120-121
racial segregation, 108
Medicare, 133, 137, 140
Medulla, 29, 31, 33, 168
epinephrine, 27, 37, 39, 80, 172, 174
norepinephrine, 27, 37, 66, 74, 172, 174
Men, *see* Gender factors
Mental illness, 45, 51-52, 148, 165, 169, 173
children, 51
community-level factors, 92
cumulative risk, 26
dementia, 39, 65, 77, 80, 165, 173

eating disorders, 9, 75, 148, 152, 156, 157
occupational stress and, 38-39
parenting and, 29
personal ties, 74
predisease pathways, 26, 29, 32
primary prevention, 51
socioeconomic status, 103, 105
suicide, 29, 92, 106, 110, 111
see also Alcohol and drug use; Crime and criminal behavior
Methodology, *see* Research methodology
Mexican Americans, 111
Mexico, 136
Microarray chip technologies, 6, 64, 70, 166
Migration, 110
Mind/body centers, 2, 19, 55, 142, 188
Minorities, *see* Race/ethnicity; *specific groups*
Mother-child interactions, *see* Child-mother interactions; Pregnancy and prenatal development
Mortality, 17, 168-169
communicable diseases, 123-125
differential survival processes, 5, 8, 49, 50, 82, 101
environmental exposures, 17
homicide, 91, 92, 95, 106
infant, 91, 92, 93, 119, 125, 130, 134, 135
international perspectives, 135, 136
personal ties and, 75, 76, 82, 153
race/ethnicity and, 9, 106, 107, 108, 110
socioeconomic status, 91, 92, 95, 100-103 (passim), 135
suicide, 29, 92, 106, 110, 111
see also Life expectancy
Moving to Opportunity program, 93, 96
Multidisciplinary approaches, 1, 3, 4, 13-14, 18, 21-22, 179-180
committee study at hand, *xi-xii*, 19, 20, 21
community-level factors, 92-93
environmentally induced gene expression, 64, 70
interventions, 11, 12, 178-179, 187
nonlinearities, 177
personal ties, 84
positive health, 51, 56
primary prevention, 51
professional education, 3, 13, 188

N

National Cancer Act, 1, 19
National Cancer Institute, 1, 19, 157-158
National Cholesterol Education Program, 139
National Health and Nutrition Examination Survey (NHANES), 123, 185
National Health Interview Survey, 185
National Heart, Lung, and Blood Institute, 1, 19, 51, 134, 157-158
National Institute of Allergy and Infectious Diseases, 135
National Institute of Environmental Health Sciences, 134-135
National Longitudinal Survey, 185
National Long Term Care Survey, 105, 120, 133
National Survey of Black Americans, 109-110
National Survey of Families and Households, 185
National Survey of Midlife Development in the United States, 186
Native Americans, 106, 108, 155
Neurological factors, 6, 27, 31-32, 39, 171-172
    alternative medicine therapies, 142
    catecholamines, 32
    child-mother interactions, 66
    chronic stress, 6
    dopamine regulation, 32, 34, 35
    emotional regulation, 33, 77-78
    exercise and neurogenesis, 169
    occupational stress, 39
    personal ties and, 7, 76, 77-80, 84
    positive health, 5, 46-47, 55, 57, 171
    serotonergic dysfunction, 29, 30, 32, 35, 168
    substance abuse, 35
    sympathetic nervous system, 27, 29, 32, 33
    see also Allostasis and allostatic load; Brain function and structure
Norepinephrine, 27, 37, 66, 74, 172, 174
North Karelia Project, 153-154
Nutrition, 56, 128-129, 130-131
    cancer and, 129
    diabetes and, 36
    eating disorders, 9, 75, 148, 152, 156, 157
    food preservation, 130-131
    interventions, 53, 149, 151
    parenting and behavior, 31, 68-69
    personal ties, 75
    predisease pathways, 31, 34, 128-129
    primary prevention, 52, 53
    see also Weight factors

O

Occupations, *see* Employment and unemployment
Office of Behavioral and Social Sciences Research (OBSSR), xi, 2
Organization for Economic Cooperation and Development, 120
Ovarian cancer, 155

P

Pain and pain management, 50, 127, 142, 148, 151, 152
Pan American Health Organization, 135-136
Panel Study of Income Dynamics, 105, 185
Parents and parenting, 7, 28-31, 73, 74-75
    cardiovascular disease and, 29
    community-level factors, 93
    disabled children and, 126, 143
    emotional factors and hypertension, 33
    intergenerational transfer of behaviors, 30, 31, 34, 67-68
    nutrition, 31, 68-69
    see also Child-mother interactions
Pathways, *see* Predisease pathways
Personal ties, 3, 6-7, 23, 73-90, 168
    adolescents, 36, 54, 74-75
    allostatic load, 83-84
    animal models, 7, 76, 77, 84
    brain development, 7, 73, 77-79, 84
    cancer and, 75, 151-153
    cardiovascular disease and, 76, 83
    children, 73-75; *see also* Child-mother interactions; Parents and parenting
    chronic disease and quality of life, 51
    epidemiology, 7, 75, 76, 82
    gender factors, 74, 75, 83; *see also* Marriage and marital status
    genetic factors, 7, 29, 65-66, 76, 77, 84
    genomics, 74
    hypertension, 75, 76

immune system and infectious diseases,
65-66, 77, 79-82, 84
individual behavior, 74-75, 82
informational resources, 75-76
interventions, 152-153
language, 73-74
longitudinal studies, 7, 8, 27, 84
mortality and, 75, 76, 82, 153
neurological factors, 7, 76, 77-80, 84
positive health, 82-84
predisease pathways, 4, 7, 25-26, 36-37
see also Familial factors; Marriage and
marital status; Parents and
parenting
Physical activity, *see* Exercise
Pituitary gland, *see* Hypothalamic-pituitary-
adrenal (HPA) axis
Population health, 3, 5, 10-11, 24, 37, 118-
147
cancer, 129, 131
children, 10, 118-119, 125-126, 133,
134-135, 136, 168
chronic diseases and disabilities, 119-
121, 126, 127, 130-133
communicable diseases, 118, 121-125,
133-134
cost factors, 126, 136-137, 139-140,
142, 143, 144, 153-154
elderly persons, 10, 55, 120
environmental factors, general, 10, 118
fertility, 135
individual behavior and, 10, 11, 118, 143
international perspectives, 119, 120-121,
123, 131, 135-136, 153-154,
165-166, 185-186
interventions, general, 149, 153-154,
158; *see also "medical
interventions" below*
macroeconomy, 10, 106, 118, 131-132,
135-137, 143-144
medical interventions, 11, 118, 120-121
personal ties, 75
psychological factors, 10, 11, 118
research infrastructure, 13, 184-186,
188
research methodology, 143-144, 168,
178
social factors, 10, 11, 75, 118, 143
see also Community-level factors;
Epidemiology; Genomics;
Longitudinal studies

Positive health, *xii*, 3, 5, 6, 10, 12, 45-62
adolescents, 52, 54
alcohol abuse and, 52
animal models, 46-47, 169-170
brain development, 46-47, 171
cardiovascular, 50, 52
cancer, 52
cognitive factors, 50, 52
community-level factors, 5, 8, 57
defined, 23
emotional factors, 50-51, 52, 54-55
employment, 11, 52
environmental factors, general, 5, 54, 56
genetic factors, 5, 53, 57
individual behavior and, 5, 47, 52-53,
56, 57
longitudinal studies, 12, 13, 49, 51-52,
56
neurological factors, 5, 46-47, 55, 57,
171
personal ties, 82-84
population surveys, 143
research infrastructure, 13, 45, 47, 53,
56-57
research methodology, 12, 13, 56-57,
169-170
social factors, 5, 13, 36, 46, 47, 51, 54-
57, 187
see also Health promotion; Quality of
life; Resilience and resistance
Post-traumatic stress disorder, 37-38
Poverty, *see* Socioeconomic status
Predisease pathways, 3-5, 25-44, 56
adolescents, 29, 34-35, 36, 37
allostatic load, 20, 26-27, 35-40
cognitive factors, 26, 32
committee study methodology, 2, 23
community-level factors, 2, 39, 97
defined, 3-4, 25
emotional regulation, 29, 30, 32, 33
environmental factors, general, 4, 36-39,
25-26, 32, 36-39, 97
familial factors, 4, 25-26
genetic factors, 4-5, 26, 28, 32, 155
genomics, 69-70
individual behavior and, 3-4, 25, 32, 34-
36, 176-177
intergenerational transfer of behavior,
30, 31, 34, 67-68
longitudinal studies, 4, 40, 56, 165-167,
185

mental illness, 26, 29, 32
nutrition, 31, 34, 128-129
personal ties, 4, 7, 25-26, 36-37
psychological factors, 3-5, 25, 32-34, 38, 176, 185
regulation of emotions, 29, 30, 32, 33
research methodology, 12, 13, 49, 164, 165-170, 175, 176-177
social factors, 3-5, 26, 32, 36, 165-166, 176, 185, 186-187; *see also* *"personal ties" above*
socioeconomic hierarchies, 9, 37, 91, 92, 95, 100-104 (passim), 106, 108-109, 110-111
time horizons, 23, 25
see also Primary prevention; Risk factors
Pregnancy and prenatal development, 2, 28-32
brain development, 28
chronic maternal stress, 37
fertility, 135
gene expression and, 64-65
genomics, 28
Hispanics, 111
nutrition, 130-131
smoking, 34-35
social factors, 36
socioeconomic status, 103
substance abuse, 35
teenage, 138-139
see also Birth weight; Infants
Primary prevention, 1, 2, 5, 6, 9, 11-12, 13, 51-54, 130, 148, 149
cost of, 138-140
individual behavior, 52-53
longitudinal studies, 51-52
mental illness, 51
nutrition, 52, 53
sexually transmitted disease, 123
see also Health promotion; Public education
Priorities for Prevention Research at the NIMH, 51
Professional education, 13-14, 19
multidisciplinary approaches, 3, 13, 188
Psychological factors, 3, 10, 17-18, 22
cancer, 151, 155
cardiovascular disease, 1, 33, 34, 38, 50, 76, 152
chronic disease, 34
chronic stress, 37-38

hypertension, 1, 33, 38
immune system and infectious diseases, 33-34, 151
interventions, 11, 12, 148-149, 151-152, 156, 160
mind/body centers, 2, 19, 55, 142, 188
occupational stress, 38
population-level health and, 10, 11, 118
positive health, 5, 13, 46, 47, 50-51, 56
predisease pathways, 3-5, 25, 32-34, 38, 176, 185
primary prevention, 51
recovery from disease, 50-51
research infrastructure, 13, 185, 186-187, 188
research methodology, 12, 13, 176, 180
self-efficacy, 32-33, 52, 53, 179
socioeconomic hierarchies, 9, 101, 102, 104, 105, 106
see also Attitudes; Emotional factors; Mental illness; Personal ties; Social factors
Public education, 52-54
adolescents, 54
committee study methodology, 21
cost of, 138-139
disabled children, 126
school-based interventions, 11, 54
smoking, 35, 52
see also Educational attainment; Health promotion

Q

Quality of life, 51, 119, 139, 148
pain and pain management, 50, 127, 142, 148, 151, 152

R

Race/ethnicity, 2, 37, 106-111
alcohol and drug use, 106
allostatic loads, 97
cancer, 106, 107, 108
cardiovascular disease, 106, 108-109
employment, 108
mortality rates, 9, 106, 107, 108, 110
prenatal development, 111
resilience and resistance, 110, 111
sexually transmitted disease, 122

socioeconomic status, 100, 106-111, 155
see also specific groups
Racism and discrimination, 2, 3, 9, 23-24,
    107-110, 111
  cancer/HIV patients, discrimination, 155
  medical interventions, 108
  segregation, 9, 92, 93, 108, 111
Recovery from disease, 5, 22, 49-51, 54
  animal models, 33
  cancer, 33, 75
  cardiovascular disease, 50
  differential survival processes, 5, 8, 49,
    50, 82, 101
  emotional factors, 50-51, 75
  marital status, 75
  socioeconomic status, 48-49, 104
Religion, 111
Reproductive systems and functions, 32
  see also Pregnancy and prenatal
    development
Research infrastructure, 13-14, 24, 45, 184-
    189
  animal colonies, 6, 13, 70, 184, 186, 188
  community-level factors, 95-97, 188
  Council of Public Representatives
    (COPR), *xii*, 14-15, 53, 56
  health promotion, 13, 45
  individual behavior, 176-177, 179, 180
  integration with practice, 1, 2-3
  interventions, general, 157-158, 160
  mind/body centers, 2, 19, 55, 142, 188
  population health studies, 13, 184-186,
    188
  positive health, 13, 45, 47, 53, 56-57
  psychological factors, 13, 185, 186-187,
    188
  social factors, 13, 185, 186-187, 188
  see also Multidisciplinary approaches;
    Professional education
Research methodology, 12-13, 24, 143-144,
    164-183
  allostatic load, 27, 49, 70, 172-175, 180
  committee study at hand, *xi-xii*, 2-3, 19-21
  community-level factors, 8, 95-97, 98,
    164, 170
  environmentally induced gene
    expression, 70
  interventions, 13, 157-160, 166-167,
    178-179, 180
  neurology, 169, 171-172
  personal ties, 84, 164, 168

population health, 143-144, 168, 178
positive health, 12, 13, 56-57, 169-170
predisease pathways, 12, 13, 49, 164,
    165-170, 175, 176-177
psychological factors, 12, 13, 176, 180
social factors, 12, 13, 98, 165-166, 169,
    180
socioeconomic status, 102, 170
see also Animal models; Longitudinal
    studies; Multidisciplinary
    approaches; Population health
Resilience and resistance, 3, 5, 23, 47-49,
    55, 57, 63, 164, 169-170
  children, 48
  community-level factors, 48
  differential survival processes, 5, 8, 49,
    50, 82, 101
  microarray chip technologies, 64
  race/ethnicity, 110, 111
  socioeconomic status, 48-49, 104, 110,
    111
  see also Immune system and infectious
    diseases
Respiratory system, 29, 45, 47-48, 52, 69-
    70, 81, 126, 132
  asthma, 10, 126, 134-135, 143, 148
  lung cancer, 22, 75, 126, 132
  see also National Heart, Lung, and
    Blood Institute
Risk factors, general, 2, 4-5, 9-10, 11, 19,
    20
  co-occurring, 18, 20, 26-27
  cumulative, 9, 13, 26-27
  genetics, 64, 129-130, 149
  interventions, 12, 148, 150-160
  population-level health, 126-130
  prenatal and early, 4, 25, 28-32
  see also Allostasis and allostatic load;
    Behavior, individual;
    Environmental factors; Health
    promotion; Predisease pathways;
    Primary prevention; Public
    education; *specific risk factors
    (e.g., Smoking)*
Rural areas, 98, 108, 129

S

School-based interventions, 11, 54
Serotonergic dysfunction, 29, 30, 32, 168
  substance abuse, 35

Sexually transmitted diseases (STDs), 34, 35, 121-123, 130, 133-134, 138-139
    adolescents, 122, 138-139
    HIV/AIDS, 28, 50, 108, 122, 123
Sleep, 82-83
Smoking, 22, 29, 34, 52, 92, 126, 128, 132, 140, 150-151, 154, 155
    adolescents, 34-35, 128
    cardiovascular disease, 22, 140
    gender factors, 34, 128
    prenatal development, 34-35
    tobacco tax, 150, 154, 157
Social factors, 10, 17-18, 20, 22, 97-98
    alcohol and drug use, 36
    animal colonies, 6, 7, 13, 76, 77, 84, 170, 184, 186
    cognitive factors, 22, 74
    gene expression, 64
    interventions, 11, 12, 51, 149, 151-153, 155, 156, 157, 160
    isolation, 4, 26, 74, 75, 82-83, 149, 153, 155
    occupational stress, 38
    population-level health and, 10, 11, 75, 118, 143
    positive health, 5, 13, 36, 46, 47, 51, 54-57, 187
    predisease pathways, 3-5, 26, 32, 36, 165-166, 176, 185, 186-187
    pregnancy, 36
    recovery from disease, 50-51
    research infrastructure, 13, 185, 186-187, 188
    research methodology, 12, 13, 98, 165-166, 169, 180
    see also Child-mother interactions; Community-level factors; Cultural factors; Personal ties; Racism and discrimination
Socioeconomic status, 2, 3, 7, 9-10, 19, 23-24, 48-49, 91, 92-95, 97-98, 110-117, 143
    adolescent health, 104
    allostatic load, 48-49, 103, 104
    animal studies of social hierarchies, 9, 103
    cardiovascular disease, 101, 106
    children, 48, 103, 104, 134
    chronic diseases and disabilities, 101, 131-132
    community-level factors, 92-95, 97-98, 102-103, 106, 108
    educational attainment, 9, 100, 101, 102, 107, 108, 111, 128, 132
    historical perspectives, 100-101
    immigrants, 110
    individual behavior, 9, 102-103
    international perspectives, 101-102, 104-105, 119, 130, 131, 135-136
    interventions and, 149, 155
    life expectancy, 135, 136
    longitudinal studies, 9-10, 102, 104-106, 109-110, 111
    macroeconomy, 10, 106, 118, 131-132, 135-137, 143-144
    mental illness, 103, 105
    mortality rates, 91, 92, 95, 100-103 (passim), 135
    parenting and, 31
    positive health, 52
    predisease pathways, 9, 37, 91, 92, 95, 100-104 (passim), 106, 108-109, 110-111
    pregnancy, 103
    psychological factors, 9, 101, 102, 104, 105, 106
    race/ethnicity, 100, 106-111, 155
    recovery from disease, 48-49, 104
    resilience, 48-49, 104, 110, 111
    sexually transmitted diseases, 133
    see also Employment and unemployment
South Africa, 108
Stanford Five-City Project, 154
Stanford Three Community Study, 153-154
Stigmatization, 3, 9, 23-29, 107, 109-110, 111, 155
    see also Racism and discrimination
Substance abuse, *see* Alcohol and drug use
Suicide, 29, 92, 106, 110, 111
Surgeon General, 126, 128, 132
Survey of Income and Program Participation, 185
Sustainable Seattle project, 8, 96
Sympathetic nervous system, 27, 29, 32, 33

T

Taxation, tobacco, 150, 154, 157
Technological innovations, 12, 130, 132-133, 138, 156, 160
    animal colonies, 6, 13, 70, 184, 186, 188
    food preservation, 130-131
    geographic information systems, 97

historical perspectives, 17
managed care, 141
microarray chips, 6, 64, 70, 166
Television, 75, 102
Time horizons, 4, 22, 118
  alcohol and drug use, 4, 22, 40
  genetic factors, 22
  predisease pathways, 23, 25
  see also Longitudinal studies; Population
    health
Tobacco use, *see* Smoking
Training, *see* Health promotion; Professional
    education; Public education
Triglycerides, 33
Tuberculosis, 108, 121, 123-125, 134

U

United Kingdom, 104-105, 120, 131, 165-
    166, 186
United Nations, 135-136
Urban areas, 8, 92, 97-98
  childhood asthma, 135
  race/ethnicity, 9, 108

V

Venereal diseases, *see* Sexually transmitted
    diseases

W

Weight factors
  adults, 35, 36, 52, 53, 75, 129, 156
  birth weight, 36, 65, 91, 92, 93, 96,
    119, 125, 134, 138
  childhood obesity, 153
  eating disorders, 9, 75, 148, 152, 156,
    157
Whewell, William, 22
Whitehall II Study of the British Social
    Service, 105, 165
Wisconsin Longitudinal Study (WLS), 105,
    110, 165, 172, 185
Women, *see* Gender factors
World Health Organization, 123